first place
4health

motivated to
wellness

Tom Stephen and Ginny Starkey

Published by Gospel Light
Ventura, California, U.S.A.
www.gospellight.com
Printed in the U.S.A.

Caution: The information contained in this book is intended to be solely for
informational and educational purposes. It is assumed that the First Place 4 Health
participant will consult a medical or health professional before beginning this or
any other weight-loss or physical fitness program.

Library of Congress Cataloging-in-Publication Data
Motivated to wellness.
p. cm. — (First place 4 health Bible study series)
ISBN 978-0-8307-6134-0 (trade paper)
1. Christian women—Religious life—Textbooks. 2. Christian women—Health
and hygiene—Textbooks. 3. Christian life—Biblical teaching—Textbooks.
BV4527.M68 2011
248.4—dc23
2011041883

Rights for publishing this book outside the U.S.A. or in non-English
languages are administered by Gospel Light Worldwide, an international
not-for-profit ministry. For additional information, please visit
www.glww.org, email info@glww.org, or write to Gospel Light Worldwide,
1957 Eastman Avenue, Ventura, CA 93003, U.S.A.

To order copies of this book and other First Place 4 Health products
in bulk quantities, please contact us at 1-800-727-5223. You can also
order copies from Gospel Light at 1-800-446-7735.

contents

foreword

There are many in-depth Bible studies on the market. The First Place 4 Health Bible studies are not designed for the purpose of in-depth study, but are designed to be used in conjunction with the rest of the program to bring balance into your life. Our desire is for each member to begin having a personal quiet time with God each day. This time alone with God should include a time of prayer, Bible reading and Bible study. Having a quiet time is a daily discipline that will bring the rich rewards of balance, which is something we all need.

God bless you as you begin this exciting journey toward a balanced life. God will richly bless your efforts to give Him first place in your life. Remember Matthew 6:33: "But seek first his kingdom and his righteousness, and all these things will be given to you as well."

Carole Lewis, First Place 4 Health National Director

---

about the authors

Tom Stephen and Ginny Starkey have enjoyed more than 20 years of marriage and live in Newbury Park, California. Tom serves as the pastor at Monte Vista Presbyterian Church and facilitates a social media community called PCH Disciples, which explores prayer, compassion and humility. Ginny works as an editor and writer in the midst of caring for their children: Faith, Hope, Samuel and Daniel. Together, Tom and Ginny have written Bible study curriculums for Focus on the Family, Soul Survivor and Gospel Light Vacation Bible School. In addition to publishing *Fearless: 40 Devotions on Fear*, they have worked on many other projects with Regal Books including *Lead Vertically* by Craig Johnson and *Don't Quit Get Fit* with Vicki Heath.

introduction

First Place 4 Health is a Christ-centered health program that emphasizes balance in the physical, mental, emotional and spiritual areas of life. The First Place 4 Health program is meant to be a daily process. As we learn to keep Christ first in our lives, we will find that He is the One who satisfies our hunger and our every need.

This Bible study is designed to be used in conjunction with the First Place 4 Health program but can be beneficial for anyone interested in obtaining a balanced lifestyle. The Bible study has been created in a five-day format, with the last two days reserved for reflection on the material studied. Keep in mind that the ultimate goal of studying the Bible is not only for knowledge but also for application and a changed life. Don't feel anxious if you can't seem to find the *correct* answer. Many times, the Word will speak differently to different people, depending on where they are in their walk with God and the season of life they are experiencing. Be prepared to discuss with your fellow First Place 4 Health members what you learned that week through your study.

There are some additional components included with this study that will be helpful as you pursue the goal of giving Christ first place in every area of your life:

- **Group Prayer Request Form:** This form is at the end of each week's study. You can use this to record any special requests that might be given in class.

- **Leader Discussion Guide:** This discussion guide is provided to help the First Place 4 Health leader guide a group through this Bible study. It includes ideas for facilitating a First Place 4 Health class discussion for each week of the Bible study.

- **Two Weeks of Menu Plans with Recipes:** There are 14 days of meals, and all are interchangeable. Each day totals 1,400 to 1,500 calories and includes snacks. Instructions are given for those who need more calories. An accompanying grocery list includes items needed for each week of meals.

- **First Place 4 Health Member Survey:** Fill this out and bring it to your first meeting. This information will help your leader know your interests and talents.

- **Personal Weight and Measurement Record:** Use this form to keep a record of your weight loss. Record any loss or gain on the chart after the weigh-in at each week's meeting.

- **Weekly Prayer Partner Forms:** Fill out this form before class and place it into a basket during the class meeting. After class, you will draw out a prayer request form, and this will be your prayer partner for the week. Try to call or email the person sometime before the next class meeting to encourage that person.

- **Live It Trackers:** Your Live It Tracker is to be completed at home and turned in to your leader at your weekly First Place 4 Health meeting. The Tracker is designed to help you practice mindfulness and stay accountable with regard to your eating and exercise habits. Step-by-step instructions for how to use the Live It Tracker are provided in the *Member's Guide*.

- **Let's Count Our Miles!** A worthy goal we encourage is for you to complete 100 miles of exercise during your 12 weeks in First Place 4 Health. There are many activities listed on pages 255-256 that count toward your goal of 100 miles. When you complete a mile of activity, mark off the box listed on the Hundred Mile Club chart located on the inside of the back cover.

- **Scripture Memory Cards:** These cards have been designed so you can use them while exercising. It is suggested that you punch a hole in the upper left corner and place the cards on a ring. You may want to take the cards in the car or to work so you can practice each week's Scripture memory verse throughout the day.

- **Scripture Memory CD:** All 10 Scripture memory verses have been put to music at an exercise tempo in the CD at the back of this study. Use this CD when exercising or even when you are just driving in your car. The words of Scripture are often easier to memorize when accompanied by music.

welcome to
Motivated to Wellness

At your first group meeting for this session of First Place 4 Health, you will meet your fellow members, get an overview of your materials and find out what you can expect at weekly meetings. The majority of your class time will be spent learning about the four-sided person concept, the Live It Food Plan, and how change begins from the inside out. You will also have a chance to ask any questions about how to get the most out of First Place 4 Health. If possible, complete the Member Survey on page 205 before your first group meeting. The information that you give will help your leader tailor the next 12 weeks to the needs of the whole group.

Each weekly meeting begins with a weigh-in for members. This will allow you to track your progress over the 12-week session. Your Week One weigh-in/measurement will establish a baseline of comparison so that you can set healthy goals for this session. If you are apprehensive about weighing in every week, talk with your group leader about your concerns. He or she will have some options for you to consider that will make the weigh-in activity encouraging rather than stressful.

The day after your first meeting, begin Week Two of this Bible study. This study is a companion to *Don't Quit, Get Fit* by Vicki Heath, so you may want to read that book before beginning. This session, you and your group will discover some of the guiding principles of Scripture that will motivate you to stay fit for a lifetime. As you open yourself to the truth of Scripture and share your hopes and struggles with the members of your group during the next 12 weeks, you'll find yourself becoming the healthy child of God you are designed to be!

finding hope
to run the race

SCRIPTURE MEMORY VERSE
Blessed is the man who makes the LORD his trust, who does not look to the proud, to those who turn aside to false gods.
PSALM 40:4

By October 1941, England was disheartened by constant bombing raids. Most of the country had lost hope. In the midst of the misery and despair, a defiant voice helped the country see the possibility of victory. In his now famous speech, Winston Churchill spoke words of perseverance, saying, "Never give in, never give in, never; never; never; never—in nothing, great or small, large or petty—never give in except to convictions of honor and good sense. Never yield to force. Never yield to the apparently overwhelming might of the enemy." Churchill's strength of character and absolute faith in God's ability to triumph over evil allowed a nation in the midst of an attitude of defeat to rise up and find the hope they needed to move on to victory.

As we journey through life—through the ups and downs, the straightaways and the detours—we also need to listen to words that defy the forces that seek to destroy us. Jesus came so that we "may have life, and have it to the full" (John 10:10). Satan seeks to destroy us, but no matter what he or his minions try to do to harm us or discourage us—whether through weight loss, family matters, work or even our faith—we have the certainty of our hope. We have "a faith and knowledge resting on the hope of eternal life" (Titus 1:2). God will provide the victory.

Over the next week, we'll focus on the book of Hebrews, a letter sent to early Christians to encourage them to never give up their faith in what they knew to be true. Immerse yourself in these words of hope so that you will be motivated to keep moving toward your goals of wellness in all areas of your life!

RUN FREE
Day 1

Lord, as I begin my day, help me to keep my eyes focused on You and to live with the knowledge that I am fully loved. Amen.

The book of Hebrews was a letter written to early Christians who were being tempted to forego their newfound faith in Jesus. The writer wanted to encourage the early believers not to give in to outside pressure and turn away from Jesus. The author wanted them to not only stay the course but also to prevail as they followed God's plan for their lives. Read Hebrews 12:1-3. To what is the Christian life compared?

_____

_____

_____

_____

Just as a runner focuses on the finish line, on whom should we focus (see verse 2)?

_____

_____

_____

Why should He be our focus (see verse 2)?

_____

_____

_____

_____

In order to run the race, what must we do (see verse 1)?

_____

_____

_____

God wants us to run free. Read 1 John 1:9. How do we rid ourselves of the sin that weighs us down?

_____

_____

_____

Reread our memory verse in Psalm 40:4. What "false gods"—those things, people and/or activities that we focus on instead of God—do some people in our culture worship?

_____

_____

_____

How does focusing on things other than God hinder and entangle us?

_____

_____

_____

Read Psalm 40:1-3. When we trust God for what we need, how will God respond?

_____

_____

_____

_____

Lord Jesus, thank You for promising that when I confess my sins and turn away from those things in my life that have prevented me from following You, I will receive forgiveness and be free to run this race called life. Amen.

RUN WITH PERSEVERANCE

Lord, when I face difficult times, I know You are with me and that You will use those times to do something good. Thank You that Your grace is sufficient. Amen.

Starting something new is always exciting. Whether it's beginning a new job, deciding to follow Jesus more closely or starting the First Place 4 Health program, there is an excitement that seems to be inherent in the new activity that carries us through the first weeks. But inevitably the newness wears off, and either a difficult situation arises or boredom sets in and we need to choose whether we will keep going. Reread Hebrews 12:1-3. How are we to run the race set before us?

_____

_____

_____

_____

The word "persevere" suggests that the race is a long one and that in order to successfully finish it, we need to continue running it despite anything we may encounter along the way. Read John 16:33. What does Jesus promise will happen "in this world" to those who choose to follow Him?

_____

_____

_____

What do believers have in Jesus?

_____

_____

_____

Why, or how, is that possible? What did Jesus do?

_____

_____

_____

One of the most faithful men in the history of the Church was the apostle Paul, who brought Christianity to much of the Greek world. One might think that God would have made the race easy for Paul. After all, Paul was willing; he prayed, and he took the time to travel and share the good news. But Paul had anything but an easy time. Read 2 Timothy 3:10-12. What did Paul say would happen to those who follow Jesus (see verse 12)?

_____

_____

_____

_____

Who rescued Paul (see verse 11)?

_____

_____

_____

_____

What obstacles have you encountered as you have sought to achieve a healthy, balanced lifestyle?

_____

_____

_____

_____

What can you do to overcome each of the obstacles you mentioned?

_____

_____

_____

_____

Lord, help me to persevere and leap over the obstacles before me. I will look to You for the strength I need to move toward my goals so that I live a balanced life for You and with You. Amen.

NEVER RUN ALONE

Gracious and loving Father, as I begin this day, I am reminded that You called Your disciples friends. Thank You for being the friend who knows my greatest joys and my deepest sorrows and sticks with me anyway. Amen.

On August 28, 1782, the *Royal George* sank, killing more than 900 people. While there were many attempts to salvage the ship, it wasn't until 1839 that the first successful salvage occurred. What made this attempt successful? The use of the buddy system—it was the first time it was used in diving! We were created to do things together. The life of faith was never meant to be a solo effort. Our desire to get in shape emotionally, mentally, physically and spiritually will be fulfilled not only as we work together with God but also as we work with others. Look again at Hebrews 12:1. Who surrounds us?

_____

_____

_____

Because the verse begins with "therefore," we need to look at the Scripture passage that comes before this one. Briefly review Hebrews 11. Despite the different obstacles that these witnesses encountered, what is the one thing they all shared in common?

_____

_____

_____

Read Genesis 2:15-25. Everything in creation was good, except that the man was alone. Why do you think God said that it wasn't good for the man to be alone?

_____

_____

_____

_____

How does having someone to work with, play with and spend time with enhance our relationship with God?

_____

_____

_____

Read Philippians 2:19-24. Why was Paul appreciative of Timothy's help?

_____

_____

_____

Read Ecclesiastes 4:9-12. Why are two people together better than one person alone?

_____

_____

_____

How can other members of your First Place 4 Health group be part of your "cord" (verse 12)?

_____

_____

_____

_____

In what specific ways can you be a help to others in your First Place 4 Health group?

_____

_____

_____

_____

Lord, thank You for the people in my life who can help me move toward my goals. Help me be a strong encourager for others as well. Amen.

RUN YOUR OWN RACE

*Sovereign Lord, thank You that I can trust You completely and live
a life without fear, knowing that You are in control. Amen.*

Magazines, commercials, billboards and all sorts of advertisements continually remind us that we need to look, feel and be better. Compared to airbrushed supermodels, we all feel inadequate. How can anyone compete with that sort of "perfection"? The good news is that we don't have to do so. We don't have to race against those who look perfect or spend all of their time trying to look that way. We simply have to run *our own* race. God has given us a unique opportunity—our lives—and we need to make the most of it by running our own race. Reread Hebrews 12:1. At the end of the verse, we are encouraged to run "the race marked out for us." Why do you think this advice is necessary for Christians?

We often can waste precious time by wishing we had someone else's gifts, body, relationships or job instead of being excited about the race that God has given us. Have you ever wished you were in someone else's shoes? If so, how did that impact your ability to follow God's plan?

According to Jeremiah 29:11, what kind of plan does God have for us?

Read Romans 8:28-29. Even when we encounter troubles along the race of life, what is God doing (see verse 28)?

_____

_____

_____

_____

_____

Whose image does God want us to reflect, and why is it important to model that image for others (see verse 29)?

_____

_____

_____

_____

Read 1 Corinthians 9:24-27. How is the race a Christian runs different from the race of other runners?

_____

_____

_____

_____

How can you make your body your "slave" so that you will "not be disqualified for the prize" (verse 27)?

_____

_____

_____

_____

Lord, thank You that You've laid out a race marked specifically for me.
Help me to stay on the path You've set and not get distracted by others. Amen.

RUN FOCUSED

Dear Lord, I am easily distracted by the concerns of this world. Help me keep my eyes focused on You. I want to win the prize of eternal life with You. Amen.

Have you ever seen a dog run to its master? When the dog hears its master, it looks up, sees where the master is, and then runs toward him or her. The dog never takes its eyes off the master. In the same way, according to Hebrews 12:2, each of us is called to run with our eyes focused on Jesus and never take our eyes away from Him. When we set our eyes on Him, we will find the motivation to keep running to reach our goals. Similar to the writer of Hebrews, Paul uses race imagery to describe the Christian life. Read Philippians 3:12-14. What does Paul concentrate on doing, and why (see verse 12)?

_____

_____

_____

_____

_____

What does Paul mean by saying he forgets "what is behind" (verse 13)?

_____

_____

_____

_____

_____

What specifically must you leave behind in order to move forward on your race?

_____

_____

_____

_____

_____

What is the ultimate prize for every Christian runner (see verse 14)?

_____

_____

_____

_____

According to Hebrews 12:3, why should we be encouraged to "not grow weary or lose heart"?

_____

_____

_____

Read Hebrews 12:4-13. Just as earthly mothers and fathers teach their children to avoid destructive natural impulses by disciplining the children they love, how does God, our Father, discipline us?

_____

_____

_____

Why does God discipline us (see verses 10-11)?

_____

_____

_____

How does God's discipline help each of us run a focused race?

_____

_____

_____

_____

The Lord wants to bless you today by changing your life through discipline and by walking with you and encouraging you. God is committed to helping you become a person who is holy and righteous!

Lord, You've promised to discipline me when I turn away from the unique course You have set for my life. I know that You do this for my own good. Keep my eyes focused on You as I pursue Your best for my life. Amen.

REFLECTION AND APPLICATION

Day 6

Gracious Father, I know I'll be tempted to take the easy way out in my pursuit of a balanced and healthy lifestyle. Prepare my body, mind, heart and spirit to confront temptation and stay the course You have set for me. Amen.

Who would have guessed that after John baptized Jesus, God would lead Him into the desert to be tempted by the devil? Talk about a rough beginning! No initial healings to build His confidence or successful first sermon to strengthen His sense of call. Instead, the Holy Spirit led Him into the desert where the enemy would test Him and tempt Him to take the easy way out.

Matthew 4:1-11 and Luke 4:1-13 both record Jesus' experience in the desert in some detail. After fasting for 40 days, Jesus was extremely tired and hungry, which is right when the devil made his first move by suggesting that He turn some stones into bread. But Jesus knew that following this course would eventually lead to destruction, so instead He confronted the devil with God's Word: "It is written: 'Man does not live on bread alone.'"

The devil, not one to give up easily, then showed Jesus the whole world and told Him that he would give Him all authority to rule the world—if He would simply worship him. Again, the devil was offering a shortcut to all that would belong to Jesus anyway, but this way, Jesus wouldn't have to suffer being betrayed, being denied and dying a horrible, agonizing death. However, because Jesus knew that ultimate satisfaction comes from following God's plan and only God's plan, He confronted the temptation with the truth: "It is written: 'Worship the Lord your God and serve Him only.'"

In his third and final attempt, the devil suggested that Jesus throw Himself off the Temple so that angels would save Him and thus prove that He is God. But Jesus, trusting in God's faithfulness, again answered with Scripture: "It says: 'Do not put the Lord your God to the test.'"

The devil is still up to the same old tricks, tempting us to turn away from the race God has set for each of us. How do we stay on the right course? By following Jesus' example: know Scripture, trust God's plan, and never take our eyes off the goal.

Since you joined First Place 4 Health, in what ways have you been tempted to take the easy way out?

_____

_____

_____

_____

_____

In what ways can you (or did you) overcome each of your temptations?

_____

_____

_____

_____

Jesus, thank You for Your example of sticking to God's plan when tempted to do otherwise. Keep my eyes open to the tricks of the devil so I can continue to follow Your plan as I get fit physically, mentally, emotionally and spiritually.

Day 7 — REFLECTION AND APPLICATION

Lord, let the Holy Spirit guide my thoughts as I prepare for each new day. Fill me with the hope of heaven that I can continue on my journey to be healthy in all areas of my life. Amen.

Everyone at one time or another is tempted to lose hope. When hope is fading, however, we have a choice: We can continue to live our lives feeling discouraged and without hope, or, in our desperation, turn to the One who has the ability to change our lives. In other words, we can stop placing our focus on our own abilities (or lack of abilities) and reach out to the One who truly has the ability to alter the course of our lives.

As recorded in Luke 8, Jesus encountered three people who had lost hope: a demon-possessed man who lived isolated from everyone (see verses 26-39), a woman who had lived for 12 years with a hemorrhage that doctors had been unable to cure (see verses 43-48), and an important ruler name Jairus whose daughter died while he was seeking help (see verses 40-42,49-55). Their reasons for losing hope differed dramatically, but they all had one thing in common: they were desperate and everyone else had basically given up on them.

By the end of Luke 8, however, all three had hope of a better life. In fact, all three not only had hope for their lives but also had reason to share that hope with others. What made the difference?

Jesus.

Jesus wanted to let them (and everyone else who was watching) know that God has power over "hopeless" situations. Jesus brings life. Jesus is hope.

Jesus is available to help you as well. Whenever you feel abandoned, alone or rejected—when you are tempted to think that there is no hope for you—know that Jesus is with you today and every day. Jesus can heal you and raise you back up from whatever has befallen you. Enjoy His presence and power right now. Ask Him to touch the areas in your life that need healing. Embrace the hope that will keep you focused as you run the race God has for you.

Dear Jesus, help me to remember that You have control of my life. Remind me that it is not through my abilities but through Your power that I am able to do anything. I present my body, mind, heart and soul to You. Please speak deeply into my life in such a way that I'll never doubt the hope that I have. Amen.

Group Prayer Requests

4 first place
health

Today's Date: _____

Name	Request

Results

_____

_____

_____

_____

_____

_____

avoiding the lies and walking in the light

SCRIPTURE MEMORY VERSE
*Blessed are those who have learned to acclaim you,
who walk in the light of your presence, O LORD.*
PSALM 89:15

Have you ever tried to walk through your house at night without the lights on? You tell yourself, *I know my way around. I know where everything is. I will be okay.* But then you trip over something or bump into a wall. Without light, it is easy to become disoriented and lost, even in the most familiar settings. We can be "lost in the dark" in the daylight, as well, when we tell stories to ourselves that are tainted with falsehoods:

- *I am valuable because I am attractive.*
- *I'd be more impressive if I drove a more expensive car.*
- *I'm too busy to develop a healthy lifestyle.*
- *I have a track record of making poor choices.*
- *I'm just not capable of self-discipline.*

Jesus described such work of the enemy—who is "a liar and the father of lies" (John 8:44)—as that of a thief who "comes only to steal and kill and destroy" (John 10:10). The enemy is trying to steal our joy, deny our value and destroy our ability to experience life as God intended us to experience it. Fortunately, as believers we have a Light that illuminates the darkness of these lies. This Light cannot be extinguished. It is always available and is always able to tell us how we should go and how we should get there. That light is God.

Day 1 LIGHT AND LIFE

Lord, thank You for another day to follow You in truth. Show me any area of self-delusion or darkness in my life. Thank You for bringing light into my life.

Light is used in the Bible both literally and figuratively. Literally, light came into existence through God's creative work described in Genesis. Natural light (by its very nature, properties and effects) is necessary for our physical existence. Artificial light (candles, lamps, flashlights) is used so that we can see in the darkness.

In the Bible, light is also used figuratively as a symbol of God and Jesus, so it can signify purity and holiness. It also can mean spiritual cleanliness and can show that the Holy Spirit dwells in a person. The Word of God can be a light that shows us how to follow God (see Psalm 119:105). All in all, light brings us joy. Read John 1:1-5. With what two things is Christ linked (see verses 4-5)?

Read John 8:12. How did Jesus describe Himself and anyone who follows Him?

Read John 9. What did Jesus' disciples assume about the blind man (see verse 2)?

What reason did Jesus give for the man's blindness (see verse 3)?

_____
_____
_____
_____
_____

Why were the Pharisees upset about the healing of the blind man (see verses 16,18,24)?

_____
_____
_____
_____

What did Jesus give the blind man in addition to his physical sight (see verses 35-38)?

_____
_____
_____
_____

According to verse 39, what ill did Jesus come into the world to cure?

_____
_____
_____
_____
_____

Why were the Pharisees guilty of being blind?

_____
_____
_____
_____

What do you need to "see" to believe what you know to be the truth?

_____

_____

_____

Lord, show me any blind spots I might have in my life. I want to shed
Your light on them, so I can live in Your presence. Amen.

Day
2

LIGHT AND TRUTH

Lord, please protect me from any evil influences that would seek to destroy
me or minimize my life. Amen.

We all tell stories about ourselves. Some are true and some are not accurate. Many of the stories about us have in fact been "written" by other people. We also hear a lot of stories told by our culture. We are bombarded on a daily basis by so-called factual stories that tell us how we should define ourselves—by how we look, by what we wear and by what we do. But how do we discern what is fact from what is delusion, what is true and what is false, what has value and what is worthless? Read John 10:1-10. What image did Jesus use to describe Himself and His followers (see verse 7)?

_____

_____

_____

What is the only way to be saved and have eternal life?

_____

_____

_____

Why did Jesus come to earth (see verse 10)?

_____

_____

_____

What is it that prevents us from having life "to the full" (see verse 10)?

_____

_____

_____

What are some of the lies that the world would have us believe about a person's value?

_____

_____

_____

_____

God loves you "as is," like those stickers you sometimes see on used cars! God won't love you more if you have fuller lips or thinner hips. He won't love you more if you watch *What Not to Wear* every day and follow Clinton and Stacy's fashion tips. God won't love you more if you earn a six-figure salary. He loves you *just as you are,* and He wants you to live in truth and freedom, not delusion and slavery. However, it is so easy to believe the old familiar lies. What are some of the lies you have believed—lies that have prevented you from living life "to the full"?

_____

_____

_____

_____

Read 1 Samuel 16:7. What does God value?

_____

_____

_____

Lord, help me to walk in the freedom of Your truth. Show me any areas where I may have been deceived into believing Satan's lies. Shine Your light on them and free me to live the abundant life You have for me. Amen.

LIGHT AND LOVE

Lord, in my head I know that You love me, but sometimes in my heart I feel as if I don't deserve it. Please help me to understand and accept Your love. Amen.

The Bible tells us that God, who "is light," loves us (1 John 1:5). Take a moment to think about how great God's love is. The Lord does not dispense His love for us sparingly. He does not give it out just when we think we deserve it. No, the Father lavishes His love on us. In fact, the quality of the love that He has for us has a quality that is like what a loving parent feels for his or her child. Now multiply that love by eternity. That's the type of love God has for us! And He wants us to receive the inheritance that He has for all who call Him Father. Read John 3:16. What prompted God to send Jesus to the earth?

What exactly did Jesus do for us?

Read 1 John 3:1. Because of God's love for us, what are we to Him?

Look up John 1:12-13. What do we have to do to earn God's love?

According to 1 John 4:16, why can we rely on God's love?

_____

_____

_____

_____

Because of God's great love for us, He made the ultimate sacrifice: the gift of His own Son. As we consider the grand story of God's love, we see that all that God is and all that He does is rooted and grounded in His love for us. It was in love that He created us. Love was at the core of calling and covenant with Abraham. Love was the reason for His covenant with all of the people of God, a faithful love that ultimately led Christ to the cross. So don't believe the lies that you are not spiritual enough, not old enough, not young enough or not worth enough! Remember the truth: You are called of God, and He has a destiny for your life.

Dear Father, help me to see myself as one of Your children. I want to inherit the eternal life that Jesus' death made possible for me. And I want to share Your love and good news with everyone in my world. Amen.

LIGHT AND COMMITMENT — Day 4

Dear Lord, teach me to live in Your light all of the time and with my whole heart. I want to serve only You. Amen.

When the ancient Israelites turned from the worship of the one true God to practice idolatry, they created figures made out of stone or other material and set them up in a prominent place. We see this early in the history of God's Chosen People when Jacob commanded everyone in his household to destroy the foreign gods they had with them—they apparently had been collecting them for some time. When God later led the Israelites from captivity in Egypt, they created a golden calf to worship in the wilderness (see Exodus 32). During the period of the judges, Gideon drew fire from his fellow townspeople when he destroyed an altar to Baal (see Judges 6).

Although today we do not create actual stone effigies of the false gods we worship, the ways in which we spend our time and where we spend our money do show whether we worship God or something else. Read Matthew 6:24. What did Jesus say about loving the world and loving God?

_____

_____

_____

_____

Read 1 Samuel 7:2-4. What did Samuel tell all of Israel to do to show that they truly repented and had returned to following the Lord?

_____

_____

_____

_____

According to the following verses, what will God do for those who are fully committed to Him?

2 Chronicles 16:9

_____

_____

_____

Psalm 37:5-6

_____

_____

_____

Proverbs 16:3

_____

_____

_____

Read Acts 5:1-11, the story of Ananias and Sapphira. Although these two professed to be committed believers and followers of Christ, what did they do with the money from the sale of the land (see verse 2)?

_____

_____

_____

What happened to them as a result (see verses 5,10)?

_____

_____

_____

What was the reaction of the people who heard what happened (see verses 5,11)?

_____

_____

_____

What might have happened to the Early Church if Ananias and Sapphira had been able to serve themselves _and_ God?

_____

_____

_____

When was a time in your life when you felt caught between the world and God? Briefly describe the situation.

_____

_____

_____

The cares of the world and the demands of a daily routine can cause us to become obsessed with the material and the temporary. To compromise our commitment to God, the enemy doesn't have to make us deceitful (like Ananias and Sapphira); he just has to make us busy! To become more like God, however, we need to live wholly dependent on God. We cannot live well by trying to please both God and the world. We must commit to His way, not our own.

> *God, help me to keep my feet firmly planted on the path You have for me. I want to stay committed to You and be a good example for others. Help me to wholeheartedly follow You. Amen.*

Day 5 LIGHT AND TRUST

> *Dear Lord, teach me to trust You with my whole heart, because You alone are worthy of 100 percent of my trust. As I come to know better and better, may I learn to trust You more and more. Amen.*

We tend to trust what we know and have confidence in our strengths. We embrace the familiar because it's easy and known. But God wants to take us beyond our current level of knowledge. He wants our faith to grow as it touches our weaknesses. As mentioned yesterday, part of committing ourselves to God in this way involves relinquishing our need to do things our way and instead submit to God's way. This is difficult to do, and we often struggle to yield the "right-of-way," but it is only by trusting God that we will learn His way really is the best way. Read John 12:35-36. In whom did Jesus say to trust, and why?

Read Proverbs 3:5-6. What are we instructed to do? What will happen when we do this?

According to John 14:1, what should we do when we feel troubled?

_____

_____

_____

According to Nahum 1:7, how does God feel about those who trust Him?

_____

_____

_____

_____

According to Jeremiah 48:7-8, what did God plan for His people in Judah, and why?

_____

_____

_____

Read Psalm 49:12-13. What happens to people who trust in themselves?

_____

_____

_____

Briefly describe a time when you tried to solve a problem without first going to God in prayer about it. What happened when you trusted only in your own resources?

_____

_____

_____

_____

Good Shepherd, I place my trust in You. You know the path I should take. Teach me to lean on Your power, not on my abilities. Amen.

REFLECTION AND APPLICATION

Father, I want to lift You up and glorify You. You are the power and the strength.
I seek what You offer: a life that is full and lavished with Your unearned favor.
I want to commit my life to You daily and walk always in Your light. Amen.

Trusting in our own strength and our own minds can cause us to doubt our decisions and our self-discipline. To handle the truth, we must understand that it's not about our mind, knowledge or cognitive skills—it's all about the mind of Christ! We don't need a college education to have the mind of Christ. To have the mind of Christ is to have a perspective that is always shaped by the sacrifice of the cross and the victory of the resurrection. God wants to share the mind of Christ with us—the sons and daughters of the kingdom! How amazing is that?

Read 1 Corinthians 2:16. Whose mind do believers have?

_____

_____

_____

According to Philippians 2:5, what are believers urged by Paul to have?

_____

_____

_____

Because as believers we have truth available to us through Jesus and through God's Word—"we have the mind of Christ"—what we allow to influence us and how we make decisions should be different from the rest of the world. Despite this, we sometimes still have trouble making good choices. Why do you think this is so?

_____

_____

_____

_____

The mind of Christ is only possible by the supernatural enlightenment of the Holy Spirit. God has prepared many remarkable things for those who love and follow Him—things that we can't discover or discern in our limited human minds. But the mind of Christ permits us to see true wisdom revealed by the Holy Spirit. What are a few specific ways that you can further develop your mind of Christ?

_____

_____

_____

_____

What are a few specific ways that you can show that you have the mind of Christ . . .

At home?

_____

_____

_____

At work?

_____

_____

_____

At your First Place 4 Health meetings?

_____

_____

_____

Dear Father, help me learn the truth and understand what You have to say to me. I want to follow the straight path You have planned for me, and I don't want to be led astray by the world. Help me to truly have the mind of Christ, so that the world sees You reflected in the way I live. Amen.

REFLECTION AND APPLICATION

Father God, I desire to know and be shaped by Your truth—from the inside out. Test my motives and my ambitions with Your truth. Show me behaviors that are out of step with You. Amen.

Reread Psalm 89:15, this week's memory verse. Now write the verse below from memory.

_____

_____

_____

_____

When we "acclaim" God in our lives, we are set free from those lies we tell about ourselves and are free to "walk in the light of [God's] presence"—to walk with God, who is "the light of the world" (John 8:12). No stumbling around. No self-delusion or denial. Just walking humbly and honestly with God. The word "acclaim" means to shout praise. When we acclaim God, we declare His worth above all else, and we exclaim this truth loudly and enthusiastically. Scripture is full of commands to praise God for His greatness and to shout joyfully (see, for example, Deuteronomy 32:3 and Psalm 66:1).

However, as our memory verse points out, we have to learn how to acclaim God. One of the best ways we can learn this is by practicing it—not only by always thanking God for every good thing He does, but also by being unafraid to show the world that we live the way God wants us to live and that we acknowledge God for everything that happens in our lives. Because we believe in Jesus, we are children of God. According to Luke 8:21, how are Jesus' family members supposed to act?

_____

_____

_____

_____

According to Philippians 4:9, what happens when we practice what we believe?

_____

_____

_____

_____

When someone asks you how you solved a problem you had or what led you down a certain pathway that turned out to be just the right thing to do, how do you answer?

_____

_____

_____

_____

_____

Do you truly feel that God has the lead role in your life? How can you better acknowledge and acclaim God?

_____

_____

_____

_____

_____

Take a few minutes today to do just this: Shout (or at least say out loud) how great you think God is, and tell Him why you think He is great. Do this either during your quiet time with God in a room by yourself or outside during your daily walk or jog.

> *Lord, You give me life and love, and You teach me how to walk in*
> *Your light. I want to acclaim You by practicing what I believe, and I*
> *want to lift You up for all the world to see. I want everyone to know*
> *how great You are. You have given me so very much. Amen.*

Group Prayer Requests

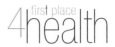

Today's Date: _____

Name	Request

Results

_____

_____

_____

_____

_____

embracing a new way of thinking

SCRIPTURE MEMORY VERSE

See, I am doing a new thing! Now it springs up; do you not perceive it?
I am making a way in the desert and streams in the wasteland.

ISAIAH 43:19

Our God is a God of the new and a God of renewal. The creation that we see all around us reflects the character of the One who created it. God is continually creating and re-creating. Cells replicate themselves, species reproduce, and new creations come into being.

You, too, are a new creation, made so by your belief in Christ. And because you are a new creation in Christ, God wants you to have a new way of thinking and viewing the world so He can continue to do more new things in your life.

God has new experiences and insights planned for each one of us that we can't see—things that will "spring up," as this week's memory verse states. There may be times when we may feel as if we are in a desert and are emotionally parched, spiritually sun-scorched, with no shade or oasis in sight. The situation looks bleak—resources are scarce and water is non-existent. But God makes a way in the desert.

We may not always see that way, but nevertheless it is there. He has also designed streams in our wasteland, and they will surface at just the right time—in His perfect timing—to nourish our parched soul and to bring us renewal.

DO NOT DWELL ON THE PAST

Father God, help me to see You as the source of renewal, of new beginnings and of second chances. Sometimes I get stuck and I focus on past failures instead of looking to You for a future and a hope. Renew my faith in You. Amen.

Have you ever done something so wrong that you felt as if you would never be forgiven? Do the consequences of mistakes in your past keep you from moving toward a brighter future? Sometimes we get so stuck in the past that we are unable to move forward. The status quo can become a death sentence for spiritual vitality.

Because of their sins, God's people were taken into captivity by the Babylonians and held in Babylonia for 70 years. After years of bondage, they probably could not imagine that the Lord would ever bring them out. But the prophet Isaiah gave them reason to hope for renewal and a return to Judah. Read Isaiah 43:14-21. What does God say He is going to do (see verses 14-15)?

_____

_____

_____

_____

Of what does God remind the people (see verses 16-17)?

_____

_____

_____

_____

Why is it important to remember what God has done in the past (see also Romans 15:4)?

_____

_____

_____

_____

What command does God give, and what does He promise (see Isaiah 43:18-19)?

_____

_____

_____

_____

Many of us often have a difficult time forgetting the past. We constantly bring up things that we have done into the present, which only serves to hamper the renewal God wants to bring into our lives. He wants us to forget these former things, just as He wanted His Chosen People to forget the sins they had committed before their captivity. Read Isaiah 65:16. When God's people turn to Him once again and are renewed, what does God say He will do about past troubles?

_____

_____

_____

_____

What are some of the consequences when someone dwells on past mistakes or hurts?

_____

_____

_____

_____

Are there things from your past that you are still dwelling on today—things that may be holding you back from complete renewal? Prayerfully ask God to show you anything you may be holding on to and instead give it to God. Clear your mind so that He can give you a new way of thinking.

Lord, create in me a refreshed mind that is focused on You and liberated from the past. Thank You for giving me a new beginning and a chance to be renewed.

DELIGHT IN THE LORD

Lord, make me cautious about the source of any advice I receive. Help me to find truth in Your Word so that I think in a right manner. May my thoughts and affections dwell only on You. You are my teacher and my delight. Amen.

"Delighting" in something can be healthy and fun—an enjoyable focus on a loved one or a hobby. If we are delighting in something, we will willingly think about it day and night. We will meditate on it. We will reflect on it. We will consider it from all angles. Just thinking about our delight makes us happier, more alive and peaceful. But can we really delight in what God says to do? Read Psalm 1:1-3. What three behaviors would prevent a person from being blessed (see verse 1)?

1. _____

2. _____

3. _____

How would a person show he or she walks "in the counsel of the wicked"?

_____

_____

_____

How would a person show that he or she stands "in the way of sinners"?

_____

_____

_____

_____

How would a person show that he or she sits "in the seat of mockers"?

_____

_____

_____

_____

In your experience with First Place 4 Health, have you been tempted to listen to "mockers" or "wicked counsel"? If so, in what ways?

_____

_____

_____

What delights someone who is blessed? On what does a blessed person meditate (see verse 2)?

_____

_____

_____

_____

What advantage does a person who does such meditation have (see verse 3)?

_____

_____

_____

Read Psalm 119:16,35. In addition to meditating, or thinking about, God's Word, what are we to do?

_____

_____

_____

_____

What can you do to remind yourself to delight in God's Word?

_____

_____

_____

_____

Lord, clear my mind of distracting thoughts and help me stay centered on You and Your Word, delighting in Your commands and following them. Amen.

BE RECONCILED WITH GOD

*Dear Lord, please make me dead to my old sinful past and alive to the new,
Spirit-driven creation that You desire me to be. Amen.*

One of the key elements of a new way of thinking is a simple decision: As
God's redeemed people, we have to decide if we are dead or alive. Are we
dead to our sinful past or not? Are we trying to nurse our weak, sinful
past back to its prior glory days of ruling our soul toward destruction,
or do we treat our flesh as dead? For new thinking—the kind that isn't
tainted by the stale toxins of the world—we need to be 100 percent dead
to the flesh and 100 percent alive to the Spirit. Read 2 Corinthians 5:16-
21. What point of view did Paul say that he once had (see verse 16)?

_____

_____

_____

_____

What changed for Paul? Why did his thinking change? (If you don't
know Paul's history, read Acts 9:1-19; 26:2-18.)

_____

_____

_____

What happens to a person who is "in Christ" (2 Corinthians 5:17)?

_____

_____

_____

What made this reconciliation possible (see verses 18-19)?

_____

_____

_____

_____

As a result, what are we to do (see verse 20)?

_____

_____

_____

_____

_____

What do we have to do to be reconciled to God—to "become the righteousness of God" (verse 21)?

_____

_____

_____

_____

Thankfully, God's process of renewal for our mind doesn't depend on our strength, faithfulness or purity. We couldn't muster enough mental energy or positive thoughts to generate a new creation within our mind—it just wouldn't happen. But when we are in Christ—when we have a faith relationship with Him—He makes it happen. What are some benefits of being "in Christ"?

_____

_____

_____

_____

It is time to bury the old and embrace what is new. What are some old habits, hang-ups or relationships that you need to let go of so that you can truly be the new creation God wants you to be?

_____

_____

_____

_____

_____

How might considering yourself to be a new creation in Christ cause you to be better able to reach your First Place 4 Health goals?

_____

_____

_____

_____

_____

Lord, help me to be reconciled to You. And help me to believe that I truly am a new creation when I believe in Jesus and all that He did for me. Thank You for the grace that You so freely give to me. Amen.

Day
4

RENEW YOUR MIND

Lord, show me any thoughts of mine that aren't true, noble or right. Teach me to filter out of my mind the worldly, impure thoughts that try to distract my focus from You. Thank you, Lord. Amen.

Each morning, many of us look forward to brewing a robust cup of coffee. However, before we can make that coffee, we first have to clean out the filter from yesterday's coffee and dump out all the dregs. If we didn't do this, the stale, old leftovers would affect the fresh pot and make the coffee taste bad. A new day deserves fresh, new coffee.

Wouldn't it be helpful if we had such a filter for our minds? If we had these "mind filters," we could stop bitter and impure thoughts from entering. We could simply catch all of these thoughts and then dump them out so they didn't affect our minds and our day going forward. Well, in a way, we *do* have a mind filter. It's God's Word. Read Philippians 4:8-9. What sort of thoughts should fill our minds (see verse 8)?

_____

_____

_____

_____

Once our minds are filled with such thoughts, what are we instructed to do (see verse 9)?

_____

_____

_____

Why are our minds so easily filled with thoughts that are wrong or distasteful or go against God's Word?

_____

_____

_____

_____

Read 2 Corinthians 10:5. What are we to do when we begin to think ungodly thoughts?

_____

_____

_____

_____

Read 1 Chronicles 28:9. While David gave his son Solomon instructions on how to build the Temple for the Lord, what instruction did he give in regard to how best to serve the Lord?

_____

_____

_____

_____

Why is it so important that we keep our thoughts pure?

_____

_____

_____

_____

How do our actions reveal what we think about God?

_____

_____

_____

_____

What have you seen in the world that you would consider true, noble, pure, lovely or admirable?

_____

_____

_____

_____

How can a person learn to think godly thoughts?

_____

_____

_____

_____

Lord, today I pray that You will make my thoughts fresh, pure and right. Raise them above the mundane and the worldly to think of You who deserve my focus and praise. Help my actions reveal Your truth and love. Amen.

Day 5 — LIVE IN THE SHADOW OF THE CROSS

Lord, as I begin a new day, give me a new understanding of the cross. Fill my mind with thoughts of Your sacrifice and Your love. Amen.

Ironically, experiencing a new way of thinking has to do with death as much as it does with life. According to this week's memory verse, we need to die to ourselves—our identity, ambition and possessions—by denying ourselves. Following Christ means walking obediently in His steps, even in the shadow of the cross. It's allowing His sacrifice to shape our thinking, our identity and our values. Read Luke 9:23-24. According to Jesus, what three things must believers do (see verse 23)?

1. _____
2. _____
3. _____

How can a person show that he or she denies himself or herself?

_____
_____
_____
_____

What does Jesus mean when He says, "Whoever wants to save his life will lose it, but whoever loses his life for me will save it" (verse 24)?

_____
_____
_____
_____

In what ways do you "lose your life" for Jesus?

_____
_____
_____

Read Romans 6:1-4. Why are believers "dead" to sin (see verses 3-4)?

_____
_____
_____

How do Christians symbolically show that they have been cleansed of their sins (see verse 4)?

_____

_____

_____

_____

Why can't we follow Christ and still hang on to our own *stuff*?

_____

_____

_____

Living in the shadow of the cross—being committed to following Christ— is a daily habit. Each day we have to die to self and let go of our preferences and seek to please God. What is most difficult about this kind of discipline for you?

_____

_____

_____

_____

Lord, today I choose to die to those behaviors that are holding me back from experiencing the fullness of the abundant life You have planned for me. I want Your sacrifice to overshadow and shape all that I do, think and value. Amen.

Day 6 — REFLECTION AND APPLICATION

Lord, I know that You want me to have a new way of thinking—one that is renewed by Your sacrifice on the cross and empowered by Your Spirit. Guide me as I develop a new way of thinking. Amen.

In Galatians 6:14-15, Paul writes, "May I never boast except in the cross of our Lord Jesus Christ, through which the world has been crucified to me, and I to the world. Neither circumcision nor uncircumcision means anything; what counts is a new creation." When you believe in Jesus, you become a new creation. Can you imagine that? You become something entirely new. You have a fresh start on your life and how you live it. Even more, you are not left alone to try to figure everything out on your own. Read Ephesians 3:14-20. This is Paul's prayer for all believers. According to verse 16, how are we strengthened?

_____

_____

_____

_____

Who dwells in our hearts? Why does God give us all of this help (see verses 17-19)?

_____

_____

_____

_____

When we ask for His help, what will Jesus do (see verse 20)?

_____

_____

_____

Starting today, make it a habit to remember that you are never alone. You don't have to make all your decisions on your own, and you don't have to worry about bad behaviors and poor decisions from the past. Because of what Christ did for you, and because of God's great love for you, you have a new way of thinking and a ready resource for the way you should go.

God, I know that You desire to reset my mind and create a fresh way of thinking in me. I ask that You would reveal any old ways of thinking that I may have so that I may be renewed and revitalized by Your Spirit. Amen.

REFLECTION AND APPLICATION

*Lord God, old hurts, habits and failures try to keep me from seeing
You and the newness that You desire to bring into my life. I believe that
You can do more than I can even imagine. Please give me the strength
today to live the way that truly honors You. Thank you, Lord. Amen.*

Reread this week's memory verse. What new things do you think God is
causing to "spring up" within you?

_____

_____

_____

_____

How do you feel about each of these new things? Excited, anxious or
confused? Why?

_____

_____

_____

_____

_____

How does knowing that God is with you reassure you?

_____

_____

_____

_____

What are the blocks in your mind that keep you from delighting in the
Lord and acknowledging that you are a new creation in Christ?

_____

_____

_____

_____

Find time today to take a prayer walk. Look for signs of newness on your walk: the growth of a flower, a recently painted house, a baby, a puppy, or something else. When you are finished with your walk, record the signs of newness you found in the space below.

_____

_____

_____

_____

_____

Thank God for each sign of newness. See it as a reminder of what He wants to do with your thinking through His grace and power.

> *I praise You, God, for Your power that is at work within me, changing the way I think and live, making me more and more like Your Son every day. Thank You for the gift of Your grace that You so freely have given me. You are and do so much more than I can even imagine. Help me to trust You more and more, and let me lean on You so that I will never be afraid. Amen.*

Group Prayer Requests

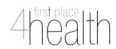

Today's Date: _____

Name	Request

Results

_____

_____

_____

_____

_____

overcoming obstacles and training for success

SCRIPTURE MEMORY VERSE

Let us not become weary in doing good, for at the proper time we will reap a harvest if we do not give up.

GALATIANS 6:9

Long-distance runners train themselves to push through the walls of pain and fatigue that entice them to quit. By training every day, these athletes discipline their bodies and their minds so that at the proper time—the time of the race—they will be equipped physically, mentally and emotionally to perform at their optimal levels.

Following Christ is like a long-distance race and requires endurance, mental fortitude, discipline and practice. Nobody gets in shape for a faith journey in a single Sunday of worship, by reading just one chapter of the Bible, by praying to God only when something bad happens.

Like athletes who train for the big race, we may also be tempted at times to quit our training for wellness and a balanced lifestyle. In the pursuit of the abundant life God has promised to us, there are a number of detours, distractions and dips in the road. But the warning in this week's memory verse is clear: We are told to "not become weary in doing good." Why would we become weary "in doing good"? Working for the Lord requires effort and energy. If our lives are out of balance, we simply can't do well what God calls us to do.

We can, however, train to do well and achieve success.

DO NOT BECOME WEARY

*Lord, train my heart to be strong and not feeble. Train my mind to be
disciplined and focused on what is good. Train my spirit to be resolute. Amen.*

Motivation is the key to not growing weary. Long-distance runners stay
focused on the goal of finishing the race. They visualize crossing the finish line and being victorious. They don't focus on any pain they may feel,
how tired they may feel, or the distance they have yet to run to reach the
finish line. They don't turn around and look at where they have been—
they just press on toward their goal. They don't lose heart. Why might
Christians become discouraged and lose heart?

_____

_____

_____

What, if anything, discourages you about reaching the goals you set for
yourself in the First Place 4 Health program?

_____

_____

Although we might think about giving up on ourselves, we *do* have reason to be encouraged and not become weary. Read Romans 8:35-39. According to verses 35 and 38-39, what cannot separate us from God's love?

_____

_____

_____

According to verse 37, what are we able to be, and why?

_____

_____

_____

_____

What specific things can you do for yourself so that you do not give up and grow faint-hearted or weary?

_____

_____

_____

_____

What specific things can you do for others in the First Place 4 Health program so that they do not become weary?

_____

_____

_____

_____

Lord, I don't want to be left by the side of the road, discouraged and weak, having lost sight of my earthly goals or my heavenly goal. Help me to run encouraged by the fact that You love me and won't give up on me. Amen.

USE YOUR TIME EFFECTIVELY

Day 2

Dear Lord, I want to invest my time wisely and not waste even one day that You have given to me. Teach me to walk with my eye on eternity. Amen.

The concept of time in this week's memory verse doesn't have to do with a measurable period but with the quality or the significance of a particular moment. In terms of a race, it has to do with running with a purpose, rather than running with great speed. It's about keeping the goal in mind as we run. How does looking at time as a particularly significant moment help motivate a runner who might grow weary over a measurable period of time?

_____

_____

_____

_____

Read Psalm 103:15. What are a person's days like?

_____

_____

_____

_____

How does Psalm 39:4-5 describe our time on earth?

_____

_____

_____

_____

Read Psalm 90:12. What should we do with our days, and why?

_____

_____

_____

_____

Look up Romans 14:12. What will we someday have to do in regard to our time on earth?

_____

_____

_____

_____

Why, then, is it important for us to gain hearts of wisdom?

_____

_____

_____

_____

God, help me to be wise in how I use the time You have given me. Teach me to invest each day with purpose and with values that reflect Your kingdom. Amen.

USE THE BUDDY SYSTEM

Day

3

Dear Lord, thank You for putting other people in my life who can help me stay on track and be stronger than I would be if I tried to go it alone. Amen.

In 1 Corinthians 12:12-31, Paul uses an analogy of the body to indicate how much we all really do need each other. We all need the different gifts and abilities that each person brings to the table. Just as a foot cannot say, "Because I am not a hand, I do not belong to the body" (verse 15), we cannot disengage from community—each of us is needed. We really can't do much for God's kingdom by ourselves, and apart from community, we don't grow very much. We can get so much more done when we work together. Read 1 John 1:6-7. Why is it so important to have fellowship with other believers?

_____

_____

_____

_____

When we are alone, we are much more at risk of telling ourselves half-truths and outright lies. We are more likely to make excuses for living an unbalanced lifestyle. How does working with someone else make this unlikely to happen?

_____

_____

_____

_____

What was a time when someone encouraged you by helping you up from a fall? Briefly describe the situation.

_____

_____

_____

_____

What are a few specific ways that you can be a buddy for a member of your First Place 4 Health group?

_____

_____

_____

_____

Read John 15:5-8. Why must Christ also be part of our "buddy system"?

_____

_____

_____

_____

Father God, thank You for weaving Your fellowship and that of my Christian friends into my life. Thank You for the encouragement and strength that You help us to have and share. Amen.

Day 4 — WITHSTAND THE BUMPS IN THE ROAD

Dear God, I know that You did not promise me a trouble-free life. But please help me when I hit a detour, distraction or dip in the road. Show me how to be strong when I feel pressured to go astray. Amen.

On your way to wellness in all areas of your life, you are bound to run into detours, distractions and dips in the road. Some of these troubles may be external—other people may try to entice you to fudge on your diet or ignore exercise for a day or two. Or the problems may be internal. If you don't see immediate results from your efforts, you may feel discouraged and want to quit. So, what should you do when you encounter bumps in the road? Read Psalm 18:1-6. How was David troubled (see verses 4-6)?

_____

_____

_____

The word "distress" accurately captures the angst and frustration many of us feel when we are trying to keep healthy habits and break unhealthy bonds. Distress is about a deep sense of pain and inner turmoil. In the Hebrew, the word refers to "narrowness of place"—the feeling as if you are in a tight and restricted space and there are few options. This is what David was feeling in this psalm. What did this cause him to do (see verse 6)?

_____

_____

_____

_____

What was God's response to David's cry (see verse 6)?

_____

_____

_____

Why was David so sure God would help him (see verses 1-2)?

_____

_____

_____

_____

Read Psalm 118:5-13. What did the psalmist do when he was troubled (see verse 5)?

_____

_____

_____

_____

Why wasn't the psalmist afraid (see verses 6-7)?

_____

_____

_____

What was God's response to the psalmist's cry (see verse 13)?

_____

_____

_____

_____

Why is it better to place our trust in the Lord rather than "in man" or "in princes" (verses 8-9)?

_____

_____

_____

_____

According to verse 12, the psalmist "cut [his enemies] off." As you think about your goals for wellness, what does triumphing over your enemies look like for you?

_____

_____

_____

_____

Almighty God, I praise You for Your faithful presence with me. Please remind me that when I have any problem at all, I should cry out to You. You alone are my refuge, and I know that You will answer my cry. Amen.

Day
5

BE ZEALOUS FOR THE LORD

Lord, there are many things calling for my passion and focus. Please create in me an intensity and passion to serve You alone. Amen.

True sports fans are intense. They don't change allegiances in the middle of the game or even in the middle of a losing season. These fans are often so passionate about their team that they paint their faces in the team colors and don extreme costumes. They remain loyal no matter what—just consider how successful you would be if you tried to convince them that their team was going to lose, so they might as well root for the other team. In effect, that is what Christ calls us to do. We have to become *His* devoted fans and exhibit that same unwavering passion. Read Romans 12:11-12. What are you instructed to keep (see verse 11)?

_____

_____

_____

_____

How does spiritual fervor and zeal help you not quit your wellness routine?

_____

_____

_____

_____

What three things are believers instructed to do (see verse 12)?

1. _____

2. _____

3. _____

How does hope generate joy? How would joy contribute to zeal?

_____

_____

_____

_____

Why should a believer be "patient in affliction"?

_____

_____

_____

_____

Read Psalm 119:65-72. Why does the psalmist feel that affliction is good (see verses 67,71)?

_____

_____

_____

_____

Read James 5:13-16. Under what circumstances should a believer pray (see verses 13-15)?

_____

_____

_____

_____

How effective is prayer (see verse 16)?

_____

_____

_____

_____

Lord, I want to be zealous for You—to be enthusiastic, passionate and eager to serve. Help me to become more joyful, more hopeful and always prayerful.

Day 6

REFLECTION AND APPLICATION

Lord, I call on Your unlimited strength to give me the perseverance to hang in there and not quit. I want to stay strong and not give up in doing good. Amen.

According to this week's memory verse, we are to be untiring in our efforts to do good. But exactly what is good? And who determines what is good?

Let's look at the second question first. According to the Bible, God is the One who decides what is good. We do not have the understanding or intelligence God has, and we are too easily distracted by anything and everything Satan or his minions use to catch our eyes and try to lead us away from our goals. We humans also seem to concentrate on outward appearances, while God looks at our hearts. So what we think is good is not necessarily what God thinks is good.

How do we find out what God thinks is good? Read Acts 17:11. What did the Bereans do when they wanted to find out whether what Paul said was true?

_____

_____

_____

_____

Read 2 Timothy 3:16-17. Why is the Bible an excellent authority?

_____

_____

_____

Although the Bible is our primary source for learning what God considers good, what other sources are available to us for helpful information and insight?

_____

_____

_____

_____

What are some of the things that the world considers good but that God would probably not regard the same way?

_____

_____

_____

_____

What are some of the things that you do that you think God would regard as good?

_____

_____

_____

_____

As you go about your day, try to imagine everything you do and see from God's perspective. How do you think God would evaluate your day and your activities? Would He see you doing good?

> *Dear God, help me to discern what is right and to understand all that You breathed into Your Word. Teach me to follow Your ways and viewpoint. Amen.*

Day
7

REFLECTION AND APPLICATION

Lord, I know that if I do not get tired of doing what You tell me is good, I will gather a good harvest. Help me to be committed to letting Your Word shape my motivation and my will to succeed. Amen.

This week's memory verse tells us that at the right moment, "we will reap a harvest." The word "harvest" can mean several different things: the season for gathering in agricultural crops, a mature crop, or an accumulated store or productive result. What do you think is the harvest that each believer will reap?

_____

_____

_____

What do you think the harvest looks like in the kingdom of God?

_____

_____

_____

_____

The harvest may also refer to the fruit of growth within a believer, the righteousness that grows in those who don't quit and who live God's way in the power of His Spirit. Where would you like to see growth in your life?

_____

_____

_____

_____

_____

What can you do today to cultivate the soil or to water your soul so that you can prepare for the harvest?

_____

_____

_____

_____

_____

Lord, use Your Word to train me so I have success in all my goals. You are my light and inspiration, my source of power when I feel weak and tired. I want to harvest righteousness and eternal life, and I want to help others see Your love so there will be a growing multitude of souls for You to harvest when You return. I want others to see Your love and Your goodness in everything I do. Amen.

Group Prayer Requests

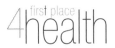

Today's Date: _____

Name	Request

Results

_____

_____

_____

_____

_____

sustaining motivation from the Word of God

SCRIPTURE MEMORY VERSE
*My eyes stay open through the watches of the night,
that I may meditate on your promises.*
PSALM 119:148

What do you do in the stillness at 2:00 AM when you can't sleep due to the pressures of the day or the anxieties of tomorrow? Do you turn on the light and read a book? Do you get up and see what's on TV? What do you do during the day when you're "in the dark" and don't know which way to turn for answers about some problem that you're having? In the obscurity of such situations, you need the light and clarity of God's Word to guide you.

In ancient times, people didn't have electric lights or even flashlights to guide them, so they actually used to tie *lamps*—like votive candles—on their feet. The lamps would throw off just enough light for them to take one step at a time. In the same way, the Word of God can shed light on any situation. The clarity of God's Word can guide you through any sort of darkness that you may encounter—any time when you can't seem to find your way or don't know what to do.

In addition to illuminating your darkest hours, God's Word casts a light that is always present. It gives you directions for how you should live at *all times*, not just for the darkest times. God's Word will encourage you, motivate you and inspire you to be the best that you can be. All you have to do is obey God's directions and have faith in His promises.

SHINE A LIGHT ON THE DARK CORNERS

Lord God, create in me a clean and well-lit heart. Renew my spirit so that You can use me for Your glory. Amen.

It's a sad but true fact of life: kids don't like chores. Perhaps when you were younger, you were one of those children who, when your mom asked you to clean the floor, swept it with speed and abandon so you could quickly get back outside and play. Perhaps you decided to cut down the time a bit by focusing on the crumbs under the table and the high-traffic areas but skipping the corners. After all, you might have reasoned, you got the dirtiest parts of the floor—why did the corners matter?

Most of us have dark corners in our hearts where we don't want the light to shine. We figure that we have mopped around the big areas and that the corners don't matter—they are clean enough. We like our private, dark retreats where we can hide "secret" things that no one but us knows about.

But is anything a secret that we can keep God from knowing? Read Proverbs 20:27. What does God do to everyone's heart?

Sometimes we may try to justify poor behavior by excusing ourselves, saying, "I'm not that bad. I didn't mean to hurt anyone, and at least I'm not as bad as that other guy!" What are some of the excuses you've heard people use to justify poor behavior or wrong choices?

Read Proverbs 16:2. Why are the excuses we use to justify ourselves, just that—excuses?

_____

_____

_____

_____

Read Psalm 139:23-24. What does David ask God to do (see verse 23)?

_____

_____

_____

_____

Why does David want God to do this (see verse 24)?

_____

_____

_____

_____

We are ready to experience a God-sustained motivation for healthy and holy living when we stop trying to hide things and allow God's light to shine in even the darkest corners of our hearts.

> _Father of light, reveal to me the dark corners of my heart. Please bring everything into the light so that I can live in Your light. Amen._

DEVELOP SOBER JUDGMENT OF YOURSELF

Day 2

> _Lord, create in me a perspective of myself that is accurate and influenced by Your Word and grace. Amen._

What would happen if we had sobriety checks outside our churches? Not to check for alcohol (though that may be appropriate in some cases), but to check for biblical sobriety before people come into church or leave to go into the community. Biblical sobriety is having an accurate view of who we are. It is both understanding and balancing our strengths and weaknesses. The only way we can ever hope to have such an accurate self-perception—one that isn't tainted by our sinful nature—is to look at ourselves calmly and slowly, appraising ourselves against what God's Word says is the truth. Read Romans 12:3. How are we to think of ourselves?

_____

_____

_____

_____

How might a person who has a too-high view of himself or herself act?

_____

_____

_____

_____

How might someone who has a too-low view of himself or herself act?

_____

_____

_____

_____

How might a lack of sober judgment impact a relationship with others? With God?

_____

_____

_____

_____

The only reason we can ever hope to have an accurate self-perception of ourselves is because of grace. Grace allows us to have a view of ourselves that is based on truth. How does God's grace help you be truthful and accurate about yourself?

_____

_____

_____

_____

While each of us has value as an individual, we are also important because of what we can contribute to the community of believers. Read Romans 12:4-8. Why are Christians like a human body?

_____

_____

_____

_____

How does this passage shed light on what your motivations should be?

_____

_____

_____

_____

Lord, help me to be mindful of who I am in You. Help me to grow my faith so that I judge only myself and my own actions. I know that I don't need to judge myself against others or even to judge others. Amen.

LOVE GOD AND OTHERS — Day 3

Lord, I want to show You how much I appreciate what You did for me. Your love is so great that I'm not sure that I can fathom it. But I do know that I want to try to spread Your love and share Your love with everyone I meet. Amen.

It's difficult to imagine, but God loves us in spite of knowing all about us. We often try to put a spin on our sin to make Him think we are *good enough* for His love, but that never works—He knows we aren't. Regardless, God loves us so much that He doesn't just want us to be with Him now; He wants us to spend eternity with Him. Read Romans 5:6-8. For whom did Christ die (see verse 6)?

_____

_____

_____

_____

_____

When did Christ die (see verse 8)?

_____

_____

_____

_____

_____

Read Matthew 22:37-40 and Mark 12:29-31. How are we to respond to God's love for us?

_____

_____

_____

_____

_____

In what specific ways can you show that you love the Lord with . . .

All your heart?

_____

_____

_____

_____

All your soul?

_____

_____

_____

_____

_____

All your mind?

_____

_____

_____

_____

All your strength?

_____

_____

_____

_____

Genuine motivation comes from the heart. If you have a passion for God, it will show up as a sustained motivation for the things that please Him. You will think of Him with affection. You will long to be with Him and connect your soul. You will be driven to reflect on His Word and shape your mind with Scripture. How does wholehearted devotion for God motivate you?

_____

_____

_____

_____

_____

It's not enough for us to have wholehearted love for God. If our love for God is real, it will also have a huge impact on our relationships with others in our family and our community. In what specific ways can you show that you "love your neighbor as yourself" (Mark 12:33)?

_____

_____

_____

_____

In what specific ways can you show that you love your First Place 4 Health "neighbors"?

_____

_____

_____

_____

Lord, I want Your love of me to be my motivation for a lifetime of loving You and loving others as myself. May my passion for You reveal my praise of You, and may my praise reach the lives of others for Your kingdom. Amen.

Day 4

REST IN JESUS

Lord, sometimes I feel beaten down and oppressed from every side, and I am desperately in need of rest. Today, I ask that You guide me, restore me and set my feet where You want them to be. Amen.

Imagine yourself lying down on a hammock between two palm trees on a beach in Hawaii. The gentle breeze causes the hammock to sway soothingly and ushers in the sweet fragrance of plumeria blossoms mixed with the salt air. Don't you wish you had such a hammock for your soul? A *soul hammock*—a place to pull away from the demands of your family and work in order to rest and recharge.

All of us at one time or another have felt too tired or too overwhelmed to keep going and keep doing the right thing. Maybe we don't see the results we expected or we think things are not happening quickly enough. Maybe we feel overwhelmed because we have one-too-many things to do, places to go or people to see. Read Matthew 11:28-30. What does Jesus offer us?

_____
_____
_____
_____

Read John 4:10. Of what is Jesus the source?

_____
_____
_____

Read John 6:35,48,51. How does Jesus describe Himself in these verses?

_____
_____
_____
_____

Refreshed by Jesus, we can keep going on. But we aren't supposed to go on alone. In Matthew 11:29-30, the "yoke" to which Jesus refers was a device placed around the necks of two animals so the two could work together. With whom should we be yoked?

_____
_____
_____
_____

What is the advantage of two being yoked to work together?

_____
_____
_____
_____

When we are harnessed this way, what are we expected to do (see verse 29)?

_____

_____

_____

_____

Why is Jesus someone with whom it would be good to work (see verses 29-30)?

_____

_____

_____

_____

Read Hebrews 2:18. Why is Jesus sympathetic to what we feel and go through?

_____

_____

_____

_____

Lord, when I feel weary, let me rest in You. I know that You understand me. Nourish me and restore my soul. I want to have the living Water and the living Bread that only You can provide. Amen.

Day 5

VALUE YOUR BODY

Lord, I want to be healthy and honor You with my body. Help me to understand that my body is Your temple, so I need to not only take care of it but value it as well. Amen.

The first Temple built by Solomon was the first permanent building in which God's presence appeared. It was God's dwelling place. Think of the most elaborate or exquisite building you have ever been in. Now

think of what goes into keeping that gorgeous building looking so spec-
tacular. Just like a valuable building, we have maintenance to perform on
our bodies—the temple of the Holy Spirit. Read 1 Corinthians 6:19-20.
To what does Paul compare our bodies, and why?

_____

_____

_____

_____

Who owns your body? Given this fact, why are you to "honor God with
your body"?

_____

_____

_____

_____

When people visit an upscale art gallery such as the Louvre in Paris,
France, they often come away as impressed by the facility as the art. The
building was designed to showcase and enhance the art and serves to
frame it. The same should be true of us. When we choose to believe in
Christ, we no longer belong to ourselves; we belong to God. The Holy
Spirit—a gift from God—comes to live inside of us. Given this, our body
should draw attention to Christ, the true work of art within us, and
showcase Him. Based on your participation in the First Place 4 Health
program, what are some specific ways you have learned to honor God
with your body in each of the four areas of your life?

_____

_____

_____

_____

Each day, you are given the gift and task of maintaining the temple the
Lord has given you. As you clean up, remodel and redecorate your body

and soul at First Place 4 Health, enjoy the process, knowing that the outcome will be a beautiful place of worship!

> *Lord, forgive me for the times I have been negligent with the upkeep of Your dwelling place—my body. Help me to remember that I no longer belong to me and that Your Holy Spirit lives within me. Amen.*

Day 6

REFLECTION AND APPLICATION

Dear God, help me to live in such a balanced way that my life reflects my love for You and Your love for me. Help me to always look to You during those dark times when I seem to stumble about, lost and disheartened. Amen.

As revealed by Jesus, the right motivation for a lifetime of balanced living is to love God and others as you love yourself. The best way to learn how to do that is to keep your eyes on God and His Word, no matter what time of day it is or where you are in the race of life.

This week's memory verse talks about "the watches of the night." In ancient Israel, the night was divided into three watches: (1) sunset to 10 PM; (2) 10 PM to 2 AM; and (3) 2 AM to sunrise. In this verse, the psalmist is describing the fact that even at night—during the darkest hours—he thinks about God's laws. After the sun goes down and before the sun comes up, God's statutes are always on his mind.

When a person lives always mindful of God's directions, he or she is much more likely to live according to God's will, which is described in God's Word. And when a person lives according to God's will, he or she reveals faith in God's promises, which are also described in God's Word. Read Psalm 119:1-3. What three things should a person do in order to receive God's blessings?

1. _____

2. _____

3. _____

Read Psalm 119:174-176. What do God's laws provide?

_____

_____

_____

_____

Briefly describe a dark "hour" when God's Word provided what you needed to see you through the "night."

_____

_____

_____

_____

What Scripture verse do you find particularly encouraging when you need guidance?

_____

_____

_____

_____

Father God, may my love be strong and my motives pure as I seek to wholeheartedly follow Your directions for my life. I want to seek You more and more so that I can walk more closely with You and for You. Amen.

REFLECTION AND APPLICATION
Day 7

Dear Jesus, Your example of persevering despite temptations to give up—of meeting needs and healing and not getting sidetracked from Your mission—has given me a model to follow in every area of my life. Help me to be more and more like You. Amen.

Meditating on God's Word will give us a renewed perspective that is distinct from the world's perspective. We will see things as they are and understand which things are part of our mission and which are not. Clarifying our mission and gaining a vision of what a fulfilled mission looks like will help us sustain our motivation. Think about all of the ways we have discussed this week on how to use the Word of God to sustain your motivation. Based on these principles, what type of mission statement could you create to avoid obstacles and stay motivated?

_____

_____

_____

_____

Imagine that this mission statement was in place in your life. How would it change your attitude? Your behaviors?

_____

_____

_____

_____

Read Philippians 2:1-5. What kind of attitude should we as Christians have? What sort of specific actions would reveal that a person has this type of attitude?

_____

_____

_____

_____

What difference would it make in your life if you were living out your personal mission statement every day?

_____

_____

_____

_____

As you conclude this week's study, really think about how you live your life: how you treat others (both those close to you and strangers you meet), what you say to others and how you say it, how you treat yourself, how you act in public and in private. Do your actions show that you have the attitude of Jesus? Would someone who watches you see that you act out what you say you believe? Would the attitude you display as you live your life attract people to God's kingdom or turn them away?

As you pray today, thank God for all of His promises and wonderful gifts, especially the gift of Jesus and His example of how we should live. Then ask God to show you where in your life you can improve so that you more closely reflect the example Jesus gave us. Ask Him to help you live out the mission statement you created today and every day.

> *Dear Jesus, I know that I should act out what I say I believe, and I know that You gave me an example to follow. Please help me to know that I can seek You and strive to be more like You, that even when I falter and stray, You are there to pick me up and lead me back on the path I should follow. Thank You so much, Lord Jesus, for all of Your many blessings. Amen.*

Group Prayer Requests

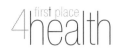

Today's Date: _____

Name	Request

Results

_____

_____

_____

_____

_____

Week Seven

living a life of worship

SCRIPTURE MEMORY VERSE
Look to the LORD and his strength; seek his face always.
PSALM 105:4

When our attention is on God, He gives us strength beyond our natural capacities. When we seek God's face, we find willpower and fortitude that we don't have when we are distracted by other things—even good things. Our attention to God, and our seeking after God, becomes our worship.

Dr. Jim Altizer, worship professor at Azusa Pacific University, defines worship as "to reflect back to God His self-revealed worth."[1] The word "worship" actually comes from the Middle English word "worthship," meaning to declare the worth of something. Worship is our way of *actively* expressing the honor, devotion and respect we feel toward God. When we worship God, we are fully engaged. Worship is also ongoing—it is not something we do only on Sundays and only in church.

Because worship gives us strength and empowers us, we can focus our minds and spirits on God's kingdom and His purpose for our lives, instead of focusing on worldly concerns and what society believes is important. And the great thing is that we can and should worship the Lord every day throughout the day wherever we are so that we are always empowered by God to do His will. We may just have to look at worship in a new way in order to take advantage of all that God has to offer us.

PRESENT A LIVING SACRIFICE

Lord, as I make choices throughout the day, help me to consider how each choice I make can be an act of worship of You. Amen.

The Old Testament contains many descriptions of the animal sacrifices the Israelites used to make as burnt offerings. There was a burnt offering (see Leviticus 6:8-13); a grain offering (see Leviticus 6:14-23); a fellowship offering (see Leviticus 7:11-13); a sin offering (see Leviticus 6:24-30); and a guilt offering (see Leviticus 5:14-19). However, in the New Testament, we are urged to make a different sort of offering. Read Romans 12:1-2. Because God is so good to us, what does Paul encourage believers to do (see verse 1)?

_____

_____

_____

"Living sacrifice" sounds like a contradiction in terms, but when we believe in Jesus, we are given a new life. Because the Holy Spirit begins to live in us, we are made alive again. By obeying God and submitting to His will, we worship God—we offer Him our bodies, minds, hearts and spirits. When we worship God with our lives, how does it change our behavior?

_____

_____

_____

How does this transformation take place (see verse 2)?

_____

_____

_____

Why is this transformation a process and not instantaneous?

_____

_____

_____

How does God's mercy impact our worship or our ability to be self-controlled and make sacrifices throughout the day (see verse 1)?

_____

_____

_____

Once we begin to renew our minds, what will we be able to do (see verse 2)?

_____

_____

_____

Read Deuteronomy 18:13. How are we to appear before God?

_____

_____

_____

Think about how you live each day. If you presented God with everything you do and say and think every day, would God find your offering acceptable and pleasing? Why or why not?

_____

_____

_____

Lord, I want You to be the center of my thoughts and service every day. In everything I do, be my focus so that I can be a worthy living sacrifice to You. Amen.

GIVE GOD FACE TIME

Day 2

Lord, You are my strength and my refuge. In You I find protection, renewal and clarity. Help me to communicate better with You so that our relationship grows closer and closer. Thank You. Amen.

In this age of digital media, face-to-face communication is becoming increasingly rare. For many of us, our "face time" is saved for just a precious few friends and family members. When we sit down with friends, it communicates that we consider them worthy of our physical presence and an investment of time. We indicate that we want to know them, understand them and have a relationship with them. They are "our people," and we want to be identified as being in relationship with them.

The same is true of God. He wants to spend time with us—personal and focused time to connect about what really matters in our lives. When we pray and give God face time, we demonstrate that we want to pursue a closer relationship with Him. He is our God, and we are His people. This communication is, in effect, another way to worship the Lord. Read Psalm 105:1-4, which contains our memory verse for this week. What does the psalmist tell believers to do as part of their worship of God?

_____

_____

_____

What are believers to seek (see verses 3-4)?

_____

_____

Read 2 Chronicles 7:14. When we seek God's face and obey God, what will He do?

_____

_____

_____

_____

Read Matthew 6:5-8. According to Jesus, how should we pray?

_____

_____

_____

_____

Why should we pray in this manner (see verse 8)?

_____

_____

_____

_____

Read Psalm 50:14-15,23. What does God want us to do?

_____

_____

_____

What will God do in return?

_____

_____

_____

According to Romans 8:26-27, what happens when we start to pray to God but don't know what to say?

_____

_____

_____

_____

Personal time with God is possible even for the busiest believer. We simply need to find God in the routine tasks of the day: riding the subway into work, waiting for a meeting to begin, standing in line for coffee or lunch, washing dishes, or pumping gas. If we can find God in the mundane, we can find Him everywhere.

Our Father in heaven, hallowed be Your name. Your kingdom come.
Your will be done on earth as it is in heaven. Give me today my daily bread.
Forgive my debts, as I have forgiven my debtors. Thank You, Lord. Amen.

MAKE A SACRIFICE

Lord God, please help me to be willing to give all of myself to You.
Help me, Lord, to hold nothing back from You. Let my life be
a sacrifice that is pleasing to You this day and every day.

A sacrifice that costs us nothing is not a sacrifice at all. A sacrifice involves giving up something—a loss of some sort. King David knew this well. In 1 Chronicles 21, David conducted a census of his soldiers in violation of a command God had given the Israelites in Exodus 30:12. In counting his soldiers, David was claiming they belonged to him and allowing pride in his nation's strength to get the best of him.

When David realized his error, he knew that he was going to have to pay a price for God to forgive the land for his sin. The Lord gave him three choices for a consequence: (1) three years of famine, (2) three months of being subject to foreign invaders, or (3) three days of plague. David replied, "Let me fall into the hands of the LORD, for his mercy is very great; but do not let me fall into the hands of men" (verse 13). Read 1 Chronicles 21:14-26. Why did David ask Araunah for his threshing floor (see verses 17-18)?

_____

_____

_____

_____

What did David want to pay for the floor (see verse 22)?

_____

_____

_____

What did Araunah want David to pay (see verse 23)?

_____

_____

_____

Why did David not accept Araunah's offer (see verse 24)?

___

Read John 15:13. What is the greatest sacrifice a person can make? What does this sort of sacrifice show?

___

According to 1 John 2:2, what did Jesus do for us?

___

God is not interested in discount sacrifices. He is not interested in merely a 10 percent tip. He is not looking for a token or a symbolic gift. He wants *all of us*. As Dietrich Bonhoeffer wrote, "When God calls a man, he calls him to die."[2] Of course, the chances of any of us being asked to give up our lives as sacrifices for anything or anyone are extremely small, but there are sacrifices we *can* make every day to show that we are willing to offer ourselves to God—to sacrifice ourselves in worship. Think over your actions of the past few days. How did you sacrifice something?

___

Lord, may each day reflect my appreciation and memory of Your great sacrificial act of love for Your people. Amen.

BECOME HOLY

Lord, set me apart for Your service, for Your glory and in Your time, not mine. Make me worthy of eternal life with You. Amen.

Worship demands wholehearted loyalty and death to anything that gets in the way of declaring the worth of God. If we want to be set apart for His service, we have to die to a self-centered life. We have to become alive to a God-centered perspective in all we do or think. And when we are sanctified, or made holy, we are set apart for a special purpose. Read 1 Thessalonians 5:23-24. What does Paul say that God promises to do for each believer?

_____

_____

_____

_____

Read Leviticus 20:7-8. Why does God want His people to be sanctified, or holy?

_____

_____

_____

According to Philippians 1:6, how can we be sure that God will sanctify us?

_____

_____

_____

_____

Read John 15:1-8. To what did Jesus compare Himself?

_____

_____

_____

_____

What are we in relation to Jesus (see verse 5)?

_____

_____

_____

Why are we already "clean" (verse 3)?

_____

_____

_____

Why is maintaining our relationship with Jesus so important?

_____

_____

_____

According to Romans 11:16, why should we consider ourselves holy?

_____

_____

_____

Being blameless does not mean that you are _perfect_. It means that you are mature and balanced. When you are "set apart," you are balanced between spirit, soul and body and have a consistent sense of integrity. You have a spirit set after God's spirit, and you demonstrate self-control and respect for your body, the temple of God. What are some specific ways that you can maintain this type of holiness?

_____

_____

_____

> _Dear Lord, I want to be set apart by You, and I want to bear much fruit for You. I never want to be separated from You. Please teach me to continually stay where I belong—with You. Thank You, Lord God. Amen._

WORSHIP IN SPIRIT AND TRUTH

Lord, center my mind on Your character as I seek to declare who You are and affirm Your preeminence in my life. Amen.

Worship centers on the character of God—who He is. To worship in spirit and truth means to focus on God as revealed in His Word. For true worship to occur, we need the proper focus (God, the source of all truth), and we need the proper approach or attitude (our spirit). We need both—truth and spirit—to worship properly. Read John 4:4-26. Why was it unusual that Jesus spoke to the woman (see verse 9)?

What did Jesus offer the woman (see verse 10)?

Why was the water that Jesus offered better than well water (see verses 13-14)?

When Jesus asked the woman about her personal life, she told Him the truth, but it was not the complete truth. What had she left out?

Jesus said that the Samaritans' worship was also not completely truthful. Why wasn't it the whole truth (see verse 22)?

_____

_____

_____

_____

What sort of worshipers does God seek? Why does He seek such worshipers (see verses 23-25)?

_____

_____

_____

_____

What did Jesus reveal about Himself (see verse 26)?

_____

_____

_____

The woman at the well was hung up on minor points of religion. She was wrapped up in function, form and location. Jesus wanted her to see the Messiah—sitting in front of her! What are some contemporary decoys we face today that keep us from seeing and worshiping Jesus?

_____

_____

_____

Read Philippians 3:3. Why is worshiping God in truth and spirit, glorifying Jesus, better than having "confidence in the flesh"?

_____

_____

_____

What is something you can do this week to enhance your worship of the Lord in spirit and truth?

_____

_____

_____

_____

_____

Dear God, help me to become a worshiper in spirit and truth. My confidence is in Your mercy and grace, not my own abilities. Only You can save. Amen.

Day 6 — REFLECTION AND APPLICATION

Lord, renew my mind with Your truth and my soul with Your Spirit so that I may worship You truthfully and faithfully in all that I do. Amen.

Worship is about giving God first place in your thoughts, affections and actions. It's looking for and interacting with God all through the day: thanking Him for your food; relating to customers, co-workers and/or friends with the attitude of Christ; and expecting God to work through you. It's focusing on Him so that you always have the strength you need for all that happens during your entire day.

Brother Lawrence lived this worship-only lifestyle. He worshiped God while he washed dishes, scrubbed floors and did other tasks. He wrote, "Let us often consider that our only business in this life is to please God."[3] Brother Lawrence had discovered a way to worship all day, in every situation. Why is it essential to understand that everything we do and say, our every act, should be done as an act of worship?

_____

_____

_____

_____

In what specific ways can you worship God in each of the four areas of your life?

Physically

_____

_____

_____

Mentally

_____

_____

_____

Emotionally

_____

_____

_____

Spiritually

_____

_____

_____

In what ways will you give God top priority this week?

_____

_____

_____

_____

_____

*Lord, help me to make worship an everyday, every way kind of thing.
I want to make my worship of You such a natural part of my life that
others will see Your hand in everything that I do and say. Amen.*

Day
7

REFLECTION AND APPLICATION

Dear God, I look to You for my strength. I want others to find You everywhere that I am. Open my eyes as I seek You, and help me to worship You in spirit and truth. Amen.

This week, we have discussed how our whole lives should be engaged in worshiping God. As we make worship the top priority in our lives, we must eliminate anything that seeks to take preeminence over Christ. True worship is only possible if we sacrifice something. He alone is worthy of our worship, and nothing else (no matter how good or noble) deserves our worship. Of course, while we need to worship God in everything we do, it doesn't mean that we should stop going to church to worship! Read Hebrews 10:24-25. What instruction does the author give?

_____

_____

_____

_____

_____

Why is worshiping with others a good thing to do?

_____

_____

_____

_____

_____

Read 1 Corinthians 12:14-20. To what does Paul compare the Church?

_____

_____

_____

_____

_____

Why is everyone in a church important to it?

_____

_____

_____

_____

_____

Remember that worshiping God brings restoration and strength—for yourself and for others. As you pray and make sacrifices of yourself, you will grow closer and closer to God and be a better reflection of Jesus, our model for how to live a balanced lifestyle. You *can* live a life of worship!

Father God, I am amazed that You seek those who seek You.
Teach me to be a good encourager so that the world sees You in all
of the loving actions of Your disciples. Amen.

Notes

1. Jim Altizer, "Worship: What, Why, How," Roadmapsforworship.com. http://road mapsforworship.com/?p=220.
2. Dietrich Bonhoeffer, *Cost of Discipleship* (New York: Collier Books, 1963), p. 99.
3. Brother Lawrence, *The Practice of the Presence of God* (New Kensington, PA: Whitaker House, 1982).

Group Prayer Requests

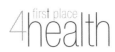

Today's Date: _____

Name	Request

Results

_____

_____

_____

_____

_____

taking time to rest

"Martha, Martha," the Lord answered, "you are worried and upset about many things, but only one thing is needed. Mary has chosen what is better, and it will not be taken away from her."

LUKE 10:41-42

In a recent study conducted by the Commission on Children at Risk, researchers found that children who are lacking in connectedness with others experience greater emotional problems, behavioral problems, academic issues, issues of substance abuse, and even medical problems such as asthma and heart disease.[1] Clearly, our brains are hardwired for relationships, and when we become too busy to connect with those we love, we pay the price.

Unfortunately, we live in a society that doesn't particularly value rest. We are a busy, driven people who feel that we must be producing something—anything—if we are to have value. As a result, we crowd our lives with activities and tasks, increasing our anxiety levels and fraying our relationships with those we love. We do better in life when we take the time to rest—just as God did and just as He intended for us to do.

Grace reminds us that God cares more about us than our performance. Not everything demands our top performance, and not everything in life is worth spending the energy, passion and time to make it excellent. Some things are worth a *good enough* effort. Such a concept will make perfectionists squirm, but when we allow ourselves to be driven by the idea that we must pursue excellence in everything and control everything to reach that goal, we only end up feeling tired, resentful and critical of others who don't share those same standards. This week, we will discover how to be effective without being hurried and how to use rest to enhance our lives.

Day 1 CHOOSE THE BETTER THING

Slow me down, Lord, so I don't run ahead of You and those with whom You want me to connect. Shape my view of time by eternity. Amen.

Studies show that 72 percent of American families with school-age children report that they don't have enough time to connect with each other, while 65 percent of working moms say they don't have enough time to relax.[2] The modern family is simply living a frazzled existence. Families are pushing to get more and more done in less and less amounts of time. As we have discussed, this type of non-stop activity comes with a cost.

In the ancient Jewish world, the concepts of time and schedules were very different. In an agrarian culture such as the one in which the Israelites lived, the time was right when the fruit was ripe. A pomegranate couldn't be hurried along—it would ripen when it was good and ready! While the farmers could pull out a calendar and tell the pomegranate that its deadline for harvest was tomorrow, they would just be wasting their breath. Interestingly, throughout the Gospels Jesus never seemed to be hurried, nor was He late. He knew how to tell time with His mission in mind.

Hospitality was also highly valued in ancient Jewish culture. In Luke 10:38-42, the Scripture passage in which our memory verse is found, we find the story of Jesus in the home of Mary and Martha. Martha, who was very concerned about being a good host, was quickly distracted by all the preparations that had to be made for her guest. Her sister, Mary, on the other hand, saw an opportunity to spend time with Jesus. What was Martha doing (see verse 40)?

_____

_____

_____

_____

_____

What was Martha's reaction (see verse 40)?

_____

_____

_____

What response did Jesus give to Martha (see verses 41-42)?

_____

_____

_____

_____

According to Jesus, why was Mary's choice better than Martha's?

_____

_____

_____

_____

_____

What do you think Jesus meant by saying, "It will not be taken away from her" (verse 42)?

_____

_____

_____

_____

When was a time in your life when you were so concerned with the details of something that you missed the bigger picture?

_____

_____

_____

_____

Notice in this story that Jesus didn't admonish or belittle Martha for her decision; He simply confronted her lovingly with the truth. Martha had confused her need to spend time with Jesus with her habit of achievement-based behavior. Mary, who took time to rest and learn from Jesus, had made the better choice.

Lord, becoming more like You means learning to tell the difference between things that are only temporary and of this world and the things that are eternal and of heaven. Teach me to always choose the better thing. Amen.

Day 2 ELIMINATE ANXIETY

Dear Lord, help me to remember to place my worries and burdens on You. Thank You, Lord God. Amen.

The frenetic pace at which we move today is a product of our culture. Magazines, websites and TV shows stress us out by telling us that we need to be constantly doing more. TV news anchors pump fear and tension into their broadcasts to maintain ratings. Talk show hosts create hype that raises our blood pressure. Everywhere we turn, we feel pressure to always have a little more—a little more effort, a little more money, a little more activity. Soon, "a little more" adds up to a whole lot.

Anxiety is created when we feel uneasy or worried about something, but don't have the resources to do anything about it. Maybe we need to solve a financial challenge, but we don't have the money to do so. Perhaps a family member is making foolish choices, but we are powerless to do anything about it. These things make us feel stuck, and we are afraid of what will happen. However, as Jesus tells us in Matthew 6:25-34, when we are a part of God's family, we really don't have to be anxious or worried about anything. According to Jesus, what should we never worry about (see verse 25)?

_____

_____

_____

In God's eyes, how do we compare with birds and flowers (see verses 26,28-30)?

_____

_____

_____

Why shouldn't we worry (see verse 32)?

_____

_____

_____

_____

What should we do instead of worrying (see verse 33)?

_____

_____

_____

_____

According to verse 27, what can worrying not do?

_____

_____

_____

_____

It is inevitable that because we are human and always try to do things on our own, at some point we will worry and become anxious about something. But according to 1 Peter 5:7, what should we do with any worry or anxiety we have, and why?

_____

_____

_____

_____

Read Psalm 94:19. When the psalmist felt anxious, what did God do?

_____

_____

_____

Today, try this simple exercise. On a sheet of paper, write down a list of all your worries and anxieties. Then talk to God about each of these items, and purposefully give each one to Him. Once you have committed these concerns into the hands of your loving heavenly Father, burn the list.

Lord, I give You all of my worries and anxious thoughts. You can handle them so much better than I can. Help me to worry less and concentrate more on seeking Your kingdom and Your righteousness. Thank You for caring about me and loving me and giving me what I need. Amen.

Day 3 FOLLOW GOD'S COMMAND

Lord, You gave us the example of resting after Your work was complete. Remind me I also need a time to rest, even if I don't think I have time for it. Amen.

Nothing in our popular culture supports the notion of the Sabbath. Leisure is big, but taking time for renewal, worship and reconnection is a rarity. Sabbath is a lost discipline for many Christians. However, it is an important part of living a spiritually and physically fit lifestyle—and it is a command from God. Read Genesis 2:1-3. After God finished creation, what did He do on the seventh day (see verse 2)?

___

On the other days, God said that what He had made was "very good." What did God do on this seventh day?

___

Read Exodus 20:8-11. What did God command us to do on the seventh day, the Sabbath (see verse 8)?

___

How are we to keep that day holy (see verse 10)?

___

According to verse 10, who is to rest?

___

According to Isaiah 56:1-8, what will God do to the person who keeps the Sabbath as instructed?

_____

_____

_____

_____

Why do you think so many people find it difficult to follow God's example and His command concerning the Sabbath?

_____

_____

_____

_____

God, help me remember Your commandment and obey it. I want to experience the many blessings You have for those who follow Your example. Amen.

Day
4

STOP THE BUSYNESS

Lord, help me to resist the pull of the world and its busyness as it tries to distract me from You and all that You offer me for my own good. Amen.

Frantic living robs us of precious energy. Some of us feel overwhelmed before we even get out of bed! Yet we know from Scripture that God never intended us to live this way. He designed both work *and* rest, setting out six days for work and one day for rest and worship. He intended this day of rest as a means for His people to relax and connect with Him. When we follow this plan, we tell God that He is the priority and our work and busyness can wait. Read Psalm 127:1-2. Who is ultimately the source of everything we have (see verse 1)?

_____

_____

_____

_____

Unless God is part of our lives, how productive are we (see verse 2)?

_____

_____

_____

_____

_____

What does God grant to those He loves (see verse 2)?

_____

_____

_____

_____

_____

Read Psalm 23:1-3. To what is God compared in this passage (see verse 1)?

_____

_____

_____

_____

Where does He lead His sheep (see verse 2)?

_____

_____

_____

_____

_____

Why are the sheep able to rest so contentedly?

_____

_____

_____

_____

_____

What happens when you stop being busy and rest with the Lord (see verse 3)?

_____

_____

_____

_____

Dear Lord, my shepherd, I know that You lead me where I need to go and that Your gifts of stillness and rest will restore me. Thank You for reminding me that all things come from You. Thank You for being with me and watching over me. Amen.

Day 5 — FOCUS ON GOD

Lord, I want to learn how to abide in You. To be at home with You, connected to Your peace and strength, so that I can remain steadfast. Amen.

Our relationship with Christ determines our fruitfulness. Throughout the day, we make decisions that cause us to remain connected with Christ or to move away from Him. Our fruitfulness depends on our intentional decision to always depend on Christ. Just as a branch detached from the vine is unfruitful, we need to maintain our union with the Source of life—the Vine, who is Christ. Read John 15:5-6. How can we gain comfort from the fact that we are the branches and Christ is the Vine?

_____

_____

_____

_____

Because God is the One who provides our day of rest, He is the One on whom we should focus during that day. By keeping the Sabbath—by resting and focusing on God—we can develop spiritual growth that activity doesn't permit. Read Isaiah 58:13-14. What does God say that we should call the Sabbath (see verse 13)?

_____

_____

_____

_____

_____

According to verse 13, what would dishonor the Sabbath?

_____

_____

_____

According to verse 14, when we honor the day of rest, what will we find?

_____

_____

_____

Read Isaiah 61:10. What reasons did Isaiah give for delighting in God?

_____

_____

_____

_____

Read Psalm 37:4. When we delight in God, what will God give us?

_____

_____

_____

_____

Think about how you usually spend your time on the Sabbath. Do you think God would be honored or dishonored by what you do? Why?

_____

_____

_____

_____

All the Bible studies we attend, sermons we hear, Christian books we read and inspirational podcasts we download are helpful, but in and of themselves they won't produce fruit in us. Only Christ can produce fruit within us—not activity. Truly, apart from Christ, we can do nothing.

Lord, I want to honor the Sabbath and delight in You. Help me to remember that I can do nothing apart from You and that the day of rest is not a day for doing as I please but as it pleases You for me to do. Amen.

Day 6 — REFLECTION AND APPLICATION

Lord, teach me to rest in You. Build my house so I don't labor in vain. Amen.

Growing personal relationships cannot be done at broadband speed, whether we are connecting with God, our spouse or our children. There is a God-designed rhythm for work and rest. Productivity is enhanced not by speed or continuous work but by a consistent pace marked by periodic breaks. In this, we need to follow the example of the good Shepherd, who leads us to safely rest in pastures and "beside quiet waters," providing the nourishment we need for restoring our souls. At the same time, as we rest with God, He will give us guidance so that we continue in the right direction. Why do you think we are more vulnerable to Satan's attacks—temptations to do wrong things or make poor choices—when we are fatigued?

_____

_____

_____

_____

Where do you feel rushed in your life?

_____

_____

_____

_____

In what specific areas of your life do you need guidance from God?

_____

_____

_____

_____

How could spending time resting and focusing on God help you to better understand what you should do?

_____

_____

_____

What are a few specific steps that you can take so that you honor God's holy day?

_____

_____

_____

_____

Shepherd God, I want to rest in You, be restored by You and be guided by You. I want to walk with You every day during the week, but on the Sabbath I want to honor and delight in only You. Help me to understand that what You want for me is good for me. Amen.

REFLECTION AND APPLICATION

Lord, I want to experience Your rest. I want others to see in me the restoration that only You can provide. Amen.

Do you want God to bless you and expand your life? If so, you need to learn God's design for Sabbath. Consider using the following R.E.S.T. acronym as a way to remember some of the principles of the Sabbath:

R   Relationships: Sabbath is for people, not production.

E   Escape the routine: Sabbath is meant to be fun and distinct from the rest of the week, so do something special on this day.

S   Spiritual: Sabbath is meant for worship, so sing, pray, meditate on God's Word and focus your attention on God.

T   Tech-free: Distractions are a hazard to Sabbath rest, so turn off the TV, computer, video games and phones for at least a few hours.

What resistance would you encounter if you suggested a weekly Sabbath at your home? How would R.E.S.T. help you benefit from the Sabbath?

On a scale of 1 to 5, with one being really bad and 5 being really good, how would you rate how you are doing in maintaining the Sabbath in your life? Why?

What steps will you implement today to consciously build a day of rest into your schedule?

_____

_____

_____

_____

What are some of the benefits of rest that you have experienced?

_____

_____

_____

_____

Rest isn't indulgent or lazy. God rested, and He designed us to need rest for a purpose—to stop our work and focus on Him. Rest makes us slow down and better able to experience and appreciate God's incredible gifts to us. Even more, when we rest, we are actually doing God's will!

> *Lord, I need to make rest a top priority in my life to connect with You and to live a lifestyle of wellness. I'm sorry that I sometimes forget just how great You are and how deserving You are of my time, my openness and my willingness to learn from You. Amen.*

Notes
1. "Hardwired to Connect—The New Scientific Case of Authoritative Communities" A Report to the Nation from the Commission on Children at Risk, Institute for American Values, Dartmouth Medical School Institute for American Values, 2003, p. 21.
2. Tim Smith, *Simple Solutions for Families in the Fast Lane* (Grand Rapids, MI: Revell, 2010), p. 26.

Group Prayer Requests

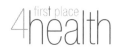

Today's Date: _____

Name	Request

Results

_____

_____

_____

_____

_____

_____

finding strength for a lifetime

SCRIPTURE MEMORY VERSE
Be strong and take heart, all you who hope in the LORD.
PSALM 31:24

At 75 years old, Jim still competes on his softball team for seniors, enjoys playing with his grandson, and regularly fishes in the surf on the beach in California. What's his secret? He says it is his growing relationship with God and his daily routine of push-ups and sit-ups. Every day he strengthens his core, both physically and spiritually.

As you pursue wellness, you will need to develop your core strength. When you strengthen your physical core—your abdominal and lower-back muscles—you will experience better balance and stability, have a greater ability to do physical activities, and more quickly reach your fitness goals. As you strengthen your spiritual core—your walk with Christ—you will have greater stability in your life, a greater ability to face any situation with confidence, and you will experience the abundant life that God desires for you.

So, how's your core? Are you walking in confidence and strength, knowing that the Lord is watching over your life? Or are you living with fear and anxiety because resources seem limited? During the next week, we will explore the lives of five "strongmen" of the Bible (Caleb, Joshua, Samson, David and Jesus) so that we can find encouragement and hope and have strength for a lifetime.

STRENGTH IN THE FACE OF OPPOSITION

*Lord, as I begin this day, open my eyes to the many truths the stories
in Your Word have to teach me. I want to be inspired and encouraged
as I learn more and more. Amen.*

It's sometimes surprising how quickly we can turn from trust and confidence in the Lord to fear and anxiety. In the story of the Exodus, the
Lord miraculously delivered His people from slavery to the Egyptians, yet
when they arrived at the border of the Promised Land, most of them
doubted God's ability to provide. Caleb was one of only two people who
stayed fast in the Lord's promises in the face of great opposition. Read
Numbers 13:17–14:10. What instructions did Moses give the spies who
were going to check out the land (see verses 17-20)?

When the spies returned to camp, they acknowledged that Canaan was
as good as the Lord had promised. However, what else did most of them
report about the land (see verses 26-29)?

What was Caleb's response to the report? How did the other spies respond to Caleb's remarks (see verses 30-33)?

What reasons did Caleb and Joshua give for taking the Promised Land (see verses 14:6-9)?

_____

_____

_____

_____

How did the people respond (see verse 10)?

_____

_____

_____

_____

On whose strength did Caleb and Joshua depend? On whose strength did the people depend?

_____

_____

_____

_____

Once the people turned away from God, He sent them back into the desert for 40 years. The adults who had rejected God's gift would never live in the "land flowing with milk and honey" (Exodus 3:8). Only Caleb and Joshua would lead the next generation into the land. Read Numbers 14:20-25. How is Caleb described? Why is this a good description (see verse 24)?

_____

_____

_____

Read Joshua 14:6-15. When the people finally entered the Promised Land after 40 years of wandering in the desert, Caleb and the rest of the people faced opposition of a different sort: There were a few areas that were difficult to conquer. When Caleb was 85 years old, what request did he make of Joshua, and why was he so sure he would be successful (see verse 12)?

_____

_____

_____

_____

_____

Although you may never face opposition on the same scale as Caleb, you may still have to confront forces that go against what you know is right or best to do. When you face opposition, what specific steps can you take to show that you are strong in your spiritual core?

_____

_____

_____

_____

_____

Gracious Lord, please give me the confidence and strength of Your servant Caleb. Help me to live my life so that my body and spirit will remain strong for a lifetime. Thank You, Lord. Amen.

Day 2

STRENGTH FOR AN IMPOSSIBLE TASK

Dear Jesus, as I consider Joshua, help me live a life that demonstrates strength and courage in the midst of seemingly impossible situations. Amen.

The Lord caused His people to wander for 40 years in the desert before bringing them to the Promised Land when Moses was 120 years old. Read Deuteronomy 34. Moses had been faced with the seemingly impossible task of leading God's Chosen People out of Egypt. What were the core spiritual strengths that he possessed that made it possible for his success (see verses 5,10-12)?

_____

_____

_____

_____

What distinguished Joshua as the next leader (see verse 9)?

_____

_____

_____

_____

Imagine not only having to take the place of one of the greatest leaders in history but also taking a group of untrained people into battle against people who were like giants and lived behind walled cities. Talk about an impossible situation! Read Joshua 1:1-9. What encouragement did the Lord give Joshua (see verses 2-5)?

_____

_____

_____

_____

In order to be successful, what was Joshua instructed to do (see verse 8)?

_____

_____

_____

Why was Joshua able to be both strong and courageous (see verse 9)?

_____

_____

_____

_____

What seemingly impossible tasks do you have in your life as you journey toward healthy living?

_____

_____

_____

_____

It often takes strength and courage to follow God's plan for your life. How do God's words to Joshua encourage you to face what seems impossible?

_____

_____

_____

_____

As you meditate on God's Word and are careful to live out the instructions that God gives in His Word, you will strengthen your core and find success.

Dear God, I choose You. I will meditate on Your promises and I will depend on Your being with me, giving me strength and courage in any situation. Amen.

Day
3

STRENGTH TO GET UP AFTER A FALL

Gracious and Holy Lord, help me to never take Your gifts for granted. Keep my eyes focused on You so that I can face temptation and turn away with resolve and joy. Amen.

In the film *Rocky Balboa,* Rocky (played by Sylvester Stallone) told his 20-year-old son, "You, me, or nobody is gonna hit as hard as life. But it ain't about how hard ya hit. It's about how hard you can get it and keep moving forward. How much you can take and keep moving forward. That's how winning is done!"[1]

Strength training includes preparing for the times when we get knocked down. In the Bible, many people were knocked down one way or another, but perhaps the most fascinating character is Samson, whose birth was announced by an angel. Read Judges 13:1-5. As Samson grew up, what impact do you think the story of his conception and birth had on his core confidence in the Lord?

_____

_____

_____

_____

Judges 14–16 tell Samson's story as a judge over Israel. In what ways did Samson prove his physical strength (see 14:6,19; 15:13-17; 16:3,25-30)?

_____

_____

_____

Why was Samson able to do such great feats of strength?

_____

_____

_____

Samson fell in love with a woman named Delilah, who was bribed by the Philistines to discover the secret of his strength. Read Judges 16:4-30. How did Samson flirt with disaster (see verses 6-14)?

_____

_____

_____

_____

Why did Samson give in to Delilah, and what was the result (see verses 15-16,19)?

_____

_____

_____

_____

After Samson lost his hair, what began to happen (see verse 22)?

_____

_____

_____

_____

What did Samson do in order to get back up after his "fall," and what was the result (see verses 28-30)?

_____

_____

_____

_____

When we confess to God a failure on our part and we ask for His help to change our behavior, He will "extend His hand" so that we can hold on to Him as we get back up. Briefly describe a time when you "fell" and thought you might never get back up. How _did_ you get back up again?

_____

_____

_____

_____

_____

Lord, thank You that I do not live life chained to past failures. I resolve to seek Your forgiveness whenever I trip up and fall. You have the strength I need to get back on my feet. Thank You for Your grace and forgiveness. Amen.

STRENGTH ON ALL OCCASIONS

Day 4

Dear Lord, as I consider the story and words of David, fill me with confidence to face any situation by trusting in Your strength. Amen.

David was a shepherd boy who was anointed king when Saul was still the ruler of Israel. David was eventually summoned to Saul's court to act as a musician, but after he defeated Goliath, Saul started to become jealous of him. David successfully completed every task that Saul gave to him, but he was eventually forced to leave the court because Saul tried to kill him. David continued to be hounded by Saul for years, and some of David's greatest psalms were written in response to what was happening to him during that time. Read Psalm 31, a prayer that David wrote when he faced a particularly dire situation and felt as if he were all alone. How does David describe what the Lord is to him (see verses 1-5)?

_____

_____

_____

_____

What does David remember about the Lord (see verses 6-8)?

_____

_____

_____

_____

After he describes his situation in verses 9-13, David tells why he believes that God will help him now. What reasons does he give (see verses 14-18)?

_____

_____

_____

_____

Although intrigue and accusations swirl around David, what does he expect from God (see verses 19-20)?

_____

_____

_____

_____

According to our memory verse (verse 24), why should we be encouraged?

_____

_____

_____

_____

Read Ephesians 6:18 and Matthew 21:22. When and how should we pray?

_____

_____

_____

_____

The best way to stay strong on all occasions is to pray every day under all circumstances and for all things, just as David did.

> *Holy and merciful Lord, thank You for being my refuge and my rock, the One I can turn to with confidence on all occasions and for all things. I will be strong and take heart today because I place all my hope in You. Amen.*

Day 5 STRENGTH THROUGH FAITH

Dear Jesus, help me to remain strong as I seek to follow You. Amen.

As you continue to strive to reach your First Place 4 Health goals, your transformation (more energy, less weight, more physical strength to pursue life, and more inner strength to face difficult days) will become noticeable to those around you, and they will probably want to know how the change occurred. At that point, you will have a choice to make. Will you simply tell them about all the sacrifice and hard work you've done during the past nine weeks? Or will you point to Christ as your source of strength?

Our success, our confidence, our inspiration, our motivation—our everything—depends on the Lord. He has been the One who has carried us when we didn't know where to turn and wanted to give up, and He is the One who will carry us long into the future as we claim His promises. Read Acts 3:1-16. What did the lame man ask for from Peter and John, and what did Peter offer to give to him (see verses 1-6)?

_____

_____

_____

_____

As Peter took the man's hand, what did the man do (see verses 7-8)?

_____

_____

_____

_____

Why was it important that Peter asked the man to walk "in the name of Jesus Christ" (see verse 6)?

_____

_____

_____

_____

Who does the man praise for his being healed (see verse 9)?

_____

_____

_____

_____

As a crowd gathered, Peter seized the opportunity to talk about what had just happened. He wanted everyone to know that God will bring healing and hope to those who call on His name. What did Peter say the man had that made him strong and led to his healing (see verse 16)?

_____

_____

_____

_____

Just calling on the name of Jesus is not enough to be assured of healing and transformation. It is when we believe that Jesus has the power—when we have faith in Him—that we can be transformed more and more into the image of God. Read 1 Peter 5:9-10. In what are we to stand firm, and why?

_____

_____

_____

_____

Dear Jesus, thank You for the promise to bring strength and restoration to my life. I commit my spirit into Your hands. Use my life as a testimony to Your power and give me the opportunity to tell others of Your love. Amen.

Day 6 · REFLECTION AND APPLICATION

God, I know that You have plans for my life—good plans. Help me to always have faith in You. With You by my side, I can face anything. I praise Your might and power. Amen.

Perhaps one of the most well-known and strong women of the twentieth century is Corrie ten Boom. Corrie grew up in a strong Christian home, never imagining how her faith would be tested and strengthened in a German concentration camp during World War II. Many times while she was in the concentration camp, she wanted to give up. However, when anger, fear and despair threatened her soul, her sister Betsie would remind Corrie of her faith and give her a new perspective on their situation.

When Betsie was near death, she had a final word of encouragement for her sister: "Corrie, your whole life has been a training for the work you are doing here in prison—and for the work you will do afterward."[2] Betsie helped Corrie to see that God was using her life and hardships to prepare her for the work she would do in the future. The Lord had a task for Corrie that extended beyond survival. After living through the terror of the Holocaust, she had an international ministry in which she spoke and encouraged others into faith and forgiveness. Her life and words proclaimed God's ability to carry people through any situation.

God wants to use your hard times and good times, your failures and your successes, to help others know Him. The work of growing strong is training for what God has for your future. And His plan is being fulfilled right now! Briefly describe a few of your past experiences that have prepared you for what you are doing right now in your life.

_____

_____

_____

_____

_____

Corrie once said, "Worry does not empty tomorrow of its sorrow; it empties today of its strength." Are worries sapping your strength today? Do you need a new perspective? If so, give thanks for what you have been given and share your concerns with God. Allow the Holy Spirit to speak a new perspective into your life.

Dear Lord, thank You for the promise to guard my heart and mind in Christ. Show me Your perspective in those areas that are weighing me down. Help me to see the plans You have for me in the future. Amen.

REFLECTION AND APPLICATION

Lord, thank You for helping to give me strength in my core—physically, mentally, emotionally and spiritually. Continue to shape and strengthen my walk with You. Amen.

When David herded sheep as a young boy, he could have never imagined that he would become one of the most significant kings in Israel's history. In the same way, when Corrie ten Boon played in her father's shop as a young child, she could have never guessed that her life would impact millions of people worldwide. Although these two individuals lived centuries apart, both David and Corrie ten Boom were strengthened by doing a couple of basic life-giving things: They meditated on God's Word and placed their hope in the Lord. Briefly describe a few people who have served as examples of strength and courage in your life.

_____

_____

_____

_____

_____

Briefly describe a few strong men and/or women who have encouraged you to walk more closely with God. What specifically about each person inspired you?

_____

_____

_____

_____

As you spend time in God's Word and set your mind on Christ in the midst of everything that happens in your life, your faith will grow stronger. You will also find that your life will become an example to help others find the strength to hope in God. Think of two people (children, family members, neighbors, someone in the missions field, and so forth) on whom you would like to have a positive and Christ-centered impact. Write down who these people are and at least one specific action you will take this week to encourage them in the Lord.

Name	Action

Lord Jesus, my faith in You continues to give me strength and hope. Let my life be a light that guides others in Your direction and into Your kingdom. Amen.

Notes

1. *Rocky Balboa*, Columbia Pictures, 2006, Internet Movie Database (IMDB). http://www.imdb.com/title/tt0479143/quotes.
2. Corrie ten Boom, *Tramp for the Lord* (Fort Washington, PA: Christian Literature Crusade, 2008), p. 11.

Group Prayer Requests

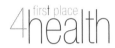

Today's Date: _____

Name	Request

Results

_____

_____

_____

_____

_____

_____

stretching for the Lord

SCRIPTURE MEMORY VERSE
*Enlarge the place of your tent, stretch your tent curtains wide,
do not hold back; lengthen your cords, strengthen your stakes.*
ISAIAH 54:2

Anne Sullivan achieved success because she remained flexible, as did her pupil, Helen Keller. Seven-year-old Helen had been blind and deaf since she was 19 months old. Twenty-year-old Anne Sullivan, who was visually impaired herself, took on the task of teaching Helen Keller how to communicate by giving Helen a doll and writing d-o-l-l in Helen's hand with her finger. As Anne gave her new objects and words, Helen's anger and frustration grew. At one point, she broke the doll and was ready to give up.

But Anne would not give up. With patience and flexibility, she tried new objects. The breakthrough came when Anne poured water over Helen's hand while spelling w-a-t-e-r on her other hand. Suddenly, Helen made the connection. The world opened up for her, and she demanded names for all the objects in her room. Helen became the first blind and deaf woman to earn a Bachelor's degree, and she eventually became an author, political activist and lecturer, inspiring millions of people. Anne Sullivan's ability to break into Helen Keller's world led her to success in her teaching. By stretching and being flexible, Helen was able to achieve what no one thought possible.

Stretching not only makes us flexible physically, but it also allows us to grow and change in ways we may once have never considered possible— in all areas of our lives.

FIND CONTENTMENT IN ALL SITUATIONS

Gracious Lord, teach me to be content in all situations. Stretch my spirit so that I trust You always with everything. Amen.

Comedian Ted Vine, who held the world record for telling the most jokes in an hour (499), once remarked, "So I said to the gym instructor, 'Can you teach me to do the splits?' He said, 'How flexible are you?' I said, 'I can't make Tuesdays.'"[1]

Often when we are asked about flexibility, we focus on what we *can't* do. We get frustrated because we haven't yet achieved our First Place 4 Health goals. We get discouraged because we still have trouble finding time to have some alone time with God. We feel disappointed in ourselves if we can't get done in one day everything we had planned to do.

Read Acts 16:16-34. As Paul and Silas sat in a prison cell, each of them had every reason to say, "I can't." They could have complained and whined about their situation, but what did they do instead (see verse 25)?

_____

_____

_____

_____

Read Philippians 4:10-13. Although Paul was happy about the gifts the Philippians had sent him, what did he say he had learned (see verses 11-12)?

_____

_____

_____

It's probably easy to understand how someone would be unhappy about being hungry or in need of the basics of life, but why do you think prosperity might also result in a person feeling unhappy?

_____

_____

_____

What is Paul's "secret" to remaining flexible despite his circumstances (see verse 13)?

_____

_____

_____

How is having a Christ-centered mindset different from simply having a positive mental attitude?

_____

_____

_____

Five words you can use to practice your flexibility are "I can because God can." As you progress on your journey with First Place 4 Health, having the attitude of being able to overcome in Christ will carry you toward your goals.

> *Lord Jesus, thank You for the ability to do all things in Your strength. Give me the ability to stretch and remain flexible as I place my trust in You. Amen.*

PERSEVERE IN ANY SITUATION   Day 2

> *Dear Lord, I want to persevere and reach my goals for a lifestyle of wellness. Help me to overcome any discouragement, any opposition, anything that tries to stop me from being the best that I can be. Amen.*

When we pursue God's best, we are called to persevere to achieve what the Lord wants for us. God calls us to stay the course. Yesterday, we saw how Paul's flexibility and contentment grew out of his relationship with Christ. However, that did not mean that Paul was complacent. Read Philippians 3:7-14. What does Paul state he wants more than anything else (see verses 8-10)?

_____

_____

_____

What was Paul's ultimate goal (see verses 11-14)?

_____

_____

_____

According to Hebrews 10:36, how do we achieve the same goal?

_____

_____

_____

Read James 1:2-4. How can troubles and problems be good things?

_____

_____

_____

What does Romans 5:3-5 have to say on the same subject?

_____

_____

_____

According to 2 Thessalonians 3:5, where did Paul hope God would direct the hearts of all believers?

_____

_____

_____

While it is true that difficult circumstances will make us stronger, ultimately God uses these situations to create a greater dependence on Him. In our weakness, we become strong through the power shown in the resurrection of Christ. God stretches us, builds our faith and blesses us when we submit to His will and live a life of perseverance.

Lord Jesus, grant me Your perspective on any difficult times I face. I am ready to receive Your power to persevere and face any challenges. Amen.

SEEK RESTORATION

God, stretch me to receive all You have for me. Create in me Your vision for my life so that I seek to live the life You have planned for me. Amen.

Walt Disney once said, "You may not realize it when it happens, but a kick in the teeth may be the best thing in the world for you." When we turn away from pursuing the Lord, sometimes we will experience difficult circumstances that end up bringing us back to God and a place of blessing.

The people of Israel experienced such difficult circumstances when God punished them for turning away from Him. When the Israelites stopped pursuing God, the Babylonians took Jerusalem and led most of the Israelites into captivity. For 70 years, they waited for deliverance. During that time, they cried out to God and developed a renewed desire to follow Him. Read Isaiah 54:1-8. To what is Jerusalem compared (see verse 1)?

_____

_____

_____

What reason do the Israelites have for singing (see verses 6-7)?

_____

_____

_____

What image in Isaiah 54:2-3 reveals that the Lord is about to give His blessing to the Israelites?

_____

_____

_____

Read Isaiah 26:15 and Isaiah 33:20. How do these verses add to the image?

_____

_____

_____

What does the psalmist ask in Psalm 51:12?

_____

_____

_____

As you have pursued wellness, how has the Lord restored your life?

_____

_____

_____

One of the greatest obstacles in the pursuit of a new life, of being restored, is fear—fear of past mistakes, fear of not being able to sustain change, fear of change itself. What does Psalm 76:6-7 say we should fear?

_____

_____

_____

The Lord wants you with Him. He wants to bless you and stretch you and restore you to your place at His side. And if God is for and with you, you have nothing to fear!

> *Gracious Redeemer, thank You for Your compassion for me.*
> *Please forgive me for those times when I went my own way and did*
> *not pursue You. Help me to live a life that honors You. Amen.*

Day 4 — REACH OUT FOR HEALING

Lord Jesus, help me to hear Your words of healing. I want to stretch and move forward in my life today. Thank You, Lord. Amen.

Long before Vicki Heath, director of leadership development for First Place 4 Health, became an author, instructor and speaker on God's call to fitness, she was a pastor's wife who felt stuck. Overweight and out of shape, Vicki felt hopeless. It wasn't until her mother-in-law encouraged her to go to a First Place 4 Health conference that she saw the possibility of change. When she saw other women in her situation who had moved out of being "stuck," it gave her hope. For the past 20 years, God has continued to stretch her by speaking into her life words of hope and strength.

Have you ever felt stuck? God wants to heal those parts of your life that hold you back from experiencing hope and health. However, He will not do it without your active participation in the process. Read Matthew 12:9-14. What did the Pharisees ask Jesus (see verse 10)?

_____

_____

_____

_____

What answer did Jesus give (see verses 11-12)?

_____

_____

_____

If you were the man with the shriveled hand, what would you have been thinking when you heard Jesus' response to the religious rulers about healing on the Sabbath?

_____

_____

_____

_____

What did Jesus tell the man to do (see verse 13), and what happened?

_____

_____

_____

_____

By stretching out his hand, what did the man show that he had?

_____

_____

_____

_____

As you reflect on your life, in what ways is the Lord calling you to stretch out your hand and to receive the healing that is waiting for you?

_____

_____

_____

_____

Are you willing to stretch out and receive all that God has for you? Are you willing to stretch out and help someone else who needs hope? If so, ask the Lord to show you the areas in your life that He wants to heal, and ask Him to show you ways to help those in need around you. Then have faith that God will do as He promises!

> *Lord Jesus, thank You for coming into my life. Heal any brokenness in me and stretch me for the plans You have for my life. Amen.*

Day 5 — FOLLOW GOD'S PLANS

Lord, create in me the ability to hear Your voice and follow Your plans. I so often design my plans and then ask for Your blessing. Help me first to seek Your plans and receive the blessings You already have in store for me. Amen.

Are you more like a reed or an oak when it comes to following God's plans? Do you flex and bend, or do you stand defiantly against the changes God wants to make in your life? There is a big difference between persevering and being stubborn. While we need to stand firm in our commitment to the Lord when storms of discouragement and despair hit, we need to pay attention to our attitude.

We often think we know what is best, so when we pray, we have a tendency to tell God what to do and how to do it. But our plans are not necessarily the same as God's. If we stubbornly stick to our agenda and are inflexible, we will not only miss God's new work but also experience unnecessary pain and suffering. Following God's will requires flexibility to bend to His will and follow where He leads.

Read Acts 10:9-48. Although the disciples had preached the gospel to other Jews, they had not planned on talking to the Gentiles about it. But then Peter had a vision. What was Peter's first, second and third reaction to the vision (see verses 14,16)?

_____

_____

_____

_____

Why did Peter feel compelled to preach the gospel to Cornelius (see verses 19-33)?

_____

_____

_____

_____

What did Peter finally realize (see verses 34-35)?

_____

_____

_____

Read Acts 16:6-10. Although Paul and his companions had planned to preach the gospel in Asia, why didn't they go there as planned (see verse 6)?

_____

_____

_____

_____

Why did the group go to Macedonia, even though it had not been part of their plan (see verse 9)? In what way did this demonstrate flexibility?

_____

_____

_____

According to Psalm 33:10-11, what are God's plans like as opposed to the plans of nations?

_____

_____

_____

According to Proverbs 19:21, how do our plans compare to God's?

_____

_____

_____

Read Isaiah 30:1. What did God say about those who carry out their own plans?

_____

_____

_____

_____

Flexibility creates opportunity. As a result of listening to the Holy Spirit, Paul and his companions launched churches in Phillipi, Athens, Ephesus, Thessalonica and Corinth. Most of Paul's letters actually came about as a result of this second missionary journey! He was flexible to God's no so that he would be open to God's yes. Are you open to being guided by the Holy Spirit even if it goes against your plans? Consider this powerful promise of God's Spirit dwelling in you: "And if the Spirit of him who raised Jesus from the dead is living in you, he who raised

Christ from the dead will also give life to your mortal bodies through his Spirit, who lives in you" (Romans 8:11).

Holy Spirit, show me Your plan for my life. If I'm headed in the wrong direction, make the way I should go clear so that I don't miss the opportunity to grow and succeed. I want to follow Your leading in all that I do. Amen.

REFLECTION AND APPLICATION

Day
6

Lord, thank You for the opportunity to love You. Create in me a flexible heart, so I can see all that You have for me. Amen.

According to the *Guinness Book of World Records,* the most flexible man in the world is Daniel Browning Smith.[2] Known as the Rubberboy, Smith can contort his body in a variety of ways because he is able to dislocate both arms and legs and turn his torso 180 degrees. He has traveled all over the world, bending in ways that seem impossible and usually shock his audiences. People are not used to seeing a fellow wrap his legs around his head!

In a similar way, most people are surprised to find someone who is flexible enough to truly love a variety of people, especially to love people who are "different." We live in a world where the first priority of most people is themselves. However, Christians are called to love others—*all* others, even our enemies—as we love ourselves. One of the greatest acts of love that we as Christians can show is to humble ourselves and place the needs of another above our own.

Read 1 Corinthians 13:4-13. As you ponder what love involves, consider how you need to flex and stretch your attitudes and actions to put the characteristics of love into practice.

When and/or with whom do you need to practice more patience and kindness (verse 4)?

What can you do to show that you are not envious, boastful or proud (see verse 4)?

_____

_____

_____

Are there particular circumstances when you have a tendency to be rude or put yourself ahead of other people (see verse 5)? If so, what can you do so that you act differently when you find yourself in those same circumstances?

_____

_____

_____

What seems to make you angry? What can you do the next time you feel yourself start to "boil" (see verse 5)?

_____

_____

_____

_____

Do you have a tendency to remember past wrongs and hurts and bring them up time and again (see verse 5)? If so, what can you do to flex and let go of the past?

_____

_____

_____

How can you show that you delight in the truth (see verse 6)?

_____

_____

_____

What do protection, trust, hope and perseverance have to do with love (see verse 7)?

_____

_____

_____

_____

Why do you think love is greater than faith and hope (see verse 13)?

_____

_____

_____

_____

Today, ask the Lord to help you stretch and become more flexible so that you can show love to each person you meet.

> *Lord, create in me a heart-attitude of love. Help me to stretch and flex with each situation I encounter so that I will show Your love to everyone I meet.*

REFLECTION AND APPLICATION

Day 7

Lord, continue to shape my heart, transform my mind and conform my will to Your desires for my life. Amen.

The first time you drive across the Golden Gate Bridge, you are impressed with its size. The bridge extends 1.7 miles from San Francisco to Marin County. The towers stand more than 740 feet above the water.

But what you don't see is even more impressive. The pillars that hold up this massive structure have been grounded approximately 220 feet below the ocean floor. Each tower alone weighs 44,000 tons. Talk about a solid foundation! And at the same time, the bridge is designed to sway more than 20 feet at the center so that when storms hit, it is flexible enough to bend without breaking. As John Maxwell writes in *Your Bridge to a Better Future,* the Golden Gate Bridge is "a beautiful example of tremendous flexibility combined masterfully with an uncompromising foundation."[3]

As Christians, we are called to remain flexible to the movement of the Holy Spirit and have the Lord as our solid foundation. This is a foundation that does not bend and shift with every new idea that comes along (see Isaiah 33:5-6) but remains firmly grounded in the Word. This strength and flexibility enables us to handle all of the storms of life that come our way without breaking and enjoy God's blessings.

Read Matthew 7:24-27, the parable of the wise and foolish builders (also told in Luke 6:46-49). Notice that the foolish builder used a foundation of sand, which fell and washed away when the winds came. The wise builder, however, used solid rock as his foundation, and his house did not fall when it was buffeted by the winds and water. In effect, it flexed but stood firm.

Flexibility in your body will come about as a direct result of stretching before and after working out. While prayer might be considered a pre-workout stretch before you begin your day, journaling about your day works much like an after-workout stretch. It gives you a chance to think about your day and remain flexible to the work that God is doing in your life. As you conclude this week's session, use the following questions to journal about what you've discovered:

In what ways have you made God the foundation of your life?

_____

_____

_____

In what ways do you show the world that God and His Word are your foundation?

_____

_____

_____

In what ways can you build on the foundation so that it continues to remain strong?

_____

_____

_____

In what ways have you felt stretched by God so that you're more flexible for what He wants to do in your life?

_____

_____

_____

As the week comes to an end, how do you feel God wants you to change so that you can fully live out His call on your life?

_____

_____

_____

_____

Dear Jesus, thank You for stretching to show me Your love and thank You for taking my hand when I stretch it out to You for help and comfort. Create in me a flexibility that allows for me to change and follow Your instructions, a flexibility that allows me to weather whatever storms come my way in life. You and You alone are my foundation. Amen.

Notes
1. Tim Vine, Famous-Quotes.com, Gledhill Enterprises, 2011. http://www.1-famous-quotes.com/quote/3544 (accessed September 2011).
2. Daniel Browning Smith, "About," *Contortionist Rubberboy.* http://www.therubberboy.com/.
3. John Maxwell, *Your Bridge to a Better Future* (Nashville, TN: Thomas Nelson, 1997), quoted in Rob Rutherford, "Flexibility from the Eagle and Turkey Parable," *On the Road from No to Go,* 2003-2011. http://www.no-to-go.com/?p=154, (accessed June 2011).

Group Prayer Requests

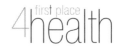

Today's Date: _____

Name	Request

Results

_____

_____

_____

_____

_____

_____

caring for your heart

SCRIPTURE MEMORY VERSE
Now devote your heart and soul to seeking the LORD your God.
1 CHRONICLES 22:19

In 1978 when the musical *Grease* stormed into theaters, a whole generation of young girls immediately identified with Sandy (played by Olivia Newton John), who falls in love with a boy from the wrong side of the tracks. Audiences wept when they heard her sing "Hopelessly Devoted to You," in which she proclaims that no matter how long it takes, she will never lose her devotion to Danny (played by John Travolta). The song quickly rose to number 3 on the Billboard Hot 100 and was even nominated for an Oscar.

Almost everyone can identify with the longing to love and be loved. God created us to have passion, which in and of itself is not a bad thing. The problem comes when we give our devotion to anyone or anything other than God, for inevitably, we will be left heartbroken. Why? Because everything of the world is temporal and fleeting. Even the best relationships will end, and eventually all things will deteriorate.

However, God is forever, and for this reason our hearts need to be fully devoted to seeking the Lord. As Jesus said, "No one can serve two masters. Either he will hate the one and love the other, or he will be devoted to the one and despise the other. You cannot serve both God and Money" (Matthew 6:24). Whether it's money, family, clothes, sports or even church, if we devote ourselves to anyone or anything other than

God, we turn away from the only One who can bring ultimate and eternal satisfaction.

This week, we will concentrate on a spiritual cardio workout. As you exercise your heart to care for it spiritually, may the Lord create in you a heart that is devoted to the One who has promised to never leave you.

Day 1 — HOPEFULLY DEVOTED

Lord, I sometimes have a divided heart. I long to know and experience Your love, but I too often find that the things of this world attract my attention away from You. Create in me a heart and soul that seek only You. Amen.

History remembers David as "a man after [the Lord's] own heart" (1 Samuel 13:14). The details of his life—the good and the bad—are recorded in the books of Samuel and Chronicles, and the psalms he wrote disclose his inner thoughts. Whether David sang in worship after experiencing God's deliverance, suffered in discouragement after the betrayal of someone close to him, or despaired with guilt over his own wrongdoing, David's passion and devotion to the Lord never waned.

In fact, he had wanted to build the Temple, the house of God, in Jerusalem. But God had a different plan in mind. Read 1 Chronicles 17:11-27. Through a revelation given to the prophet Nathan, what did David learn about his plan to build the Temple (see verses 11-12)?

_____

_____

_____

_____

Immediately after learning this news, what did David do (see verse 16)?

_____

_____

_____

In general, what did David have to say to God (see verses 16-27)?

_____

_____

_____

_____

Read 1 Chronicles 22. What did David do to set up Solomon for success in building the Temple (see verses 2-5,14-17)?

_____

_____

_____

_____

What words of encouragement did he give to Solomon (see verses 11-13)?

_____

_____

_____

_____

What did he tell the leaders of Israel to do (see verses 17-19)?

_____

_____

_____

_____

As king, Solomon set the earthly priorities for the people of Israel. But what would this act of building the Lord's Temple tell the nation and the nations surrounding Israel about who was the real ruler of Israel?

_____

_____

_____

_____

Reread our memory verse (1 Chronicles 22:19), and then read 2 Chronicles 7:14-15. What did God promise to do when His people sought His face?

Gracious and holy God, thank You that You know me. May Your Spirit work deeply in my heart so that my priorities are reshaped as necessary so that You'll be honored and glorified in what I think, say and do. Amen.

Day 2 ALWAYS YIELDING

Lord, thank You for another day to choose You. Use this time we have together to help me understand what I might be doing to create distance between us. I want to walk as closely as possible to You. Amen.

In *Finding Nemo*, a clownfish named Marlin desperately searches for his son, Nemo, who has been abducted and placed in an aquarium. A fish named Dory joins Marlin on his search, unknowingly becoming a voice of wisdom to help Marlin overcome his fears. At one point Marlin and Dory become trapped in a whale's belly, and Marlin freaks out because it appears that they are about to become lunch.

While Marlin holds on for dear life, Dory (who speaks whale) asks the creature what is happening. When she gets the response, she tells Marlin, "He says you have to let go. Everything will be okay." Marlin then asks, "How do you know—how do you know that something bad won't happen?" To which Dory replies, "I don't."

Marlin reacted like many of us do when we are faced with a situation in which we have no control. We find it hard to trust God's plan, and we want to know exactly what is going to happen. However, God calls us to yield to Him and trust Him.

In the Bible, after the Israelites had conquered the Promised Land, Joshua gathered all of the people together and asked them to consider whether they would choose to continue to follow God. Read Joshua 24:22-27. What did Joshua tell the people to throw away, and what did Joshua command them to do (see verse 23)?

_____

_____

_____

Why was (and is) a commitment to God so important?

_____

_____

_____

What did Joshua do as a sign of the people's commitment to God (see verses 26-27)?

_____

_____

_____

_____

Read Luke 22:42. Even though Jesus knew the torturous death He was facing, what did He say to show that He yielded to God?

_____

_____

_____

_____

How does knowing that even Jesus yielded to His Father's will help you yield your heart to God?

_____

_____

_____

_____

What can you do to remind yourself of your commitment to yield to
the Lord?

_____

_____

_____

_____

_____

Like the Israelites, if we don't make a commitment to place God first in
our lives, we are likely to turn away from Him. If we turn to other
"gods"—things or people that we idolize—and allow them to take hold of
our hearts, eventually we will lose both strength and life.

> *Lord, I yield my heart to You. When I am tempted to turn away from*
> *Your face, help me to turn my eyes back to You. Thank You for always*
> *pointing me in the right direction. Amen.*

Day 3

COMPLETELY GUARDED

As I begin another day, Lord, guard my heart. I confess that sometimes it can
quickly wander from Your amazing love and grace. Please forgive me. Amen.

A healthy heart is necessary for wellness in all areas of your life, and the
way to have a healthy spiritual heart is to guard it by letting God dwell
in it. Read Proverbs 4:20-23. What is the result of allowing God's wisdom to dwell in your heart?

_____

_____

_____

_____

A guard has two functions: (1) to keep some things in, and (2) to keep
other things out. Look up Galatians 5:16-26, and then make a list of

those things we should keep in our hearts and those things we should guard our hearts against.

Things to Keep In	Things to Keep Out

The apostle Paul knew the importance of guarding one's heart. Even though he was in prison when he wrote to the Philippians, he still rejoiced in the Lord's presence. Read Philippians 4:4-7. What did Paul do to keep his heart and mind under Christ as its guard?

_____

_____

_____

How can knowing that your sins are forgiven and that all of your worries are God's concern help you to feel "the peace of God" (verse 7)?

_____

_____

_____

What are a few specific things you can do to help guard your heart?

_____

_____

_____

_____

Why even during troubling times can you still experience God's peace?

_____

_____

_____

_____

Guarding your heart from outside influences may not be easy to do in our world of instant accessibility through ever-changing technology, but with the reward of God's peace waiting for you, your efforts are well worth making.

> *Lord, may the fruits of the Spirit permeate my life. Help keep my eyes steadfast on You. I want the wellspring of my life to be under Your guard. Amen.*

Day 4

CONTINUALLY MOTIVATED

Lord, thank You for giving me direction as to how to experience Your blessings. I look forward to experiencing all You have for me. Amen.

A life-sustaining motivation is the key to a long life of wholeness and health. Motivations reveal themselves in a variety of ways. Some people are naturally motivated by the desire to avoid pain. While they will never get on a treadmill for the fun of it, they will start working out after a heart attack. Other people are motivated by the benefits of exercise. The feeling they get after a great workout gives them a reason to do it all over again another day. When Moses described the Lord's plan to the people of Israel as they entered the Promised Land, he spoke both to those motivated by the desire to avoid pain and those motivated by the desire for benefits. Read Deuteronomy 28 and list the blessings that stand out to you (verses 1-14).

_____

_____

_____

_____

How would receiving these blessings strengthen your heart and trust in God?

_____

_____

_____

_____

Which painful things, or curses, seem particularly disagreeable to you (see verses 15-68)?

_____

_____

_____

_____

What impact would these negative experiences have on your ability to trust the Lord to do what He says He will do?

_____

_____

_____

_____

In order to be "the head, not the tail," what did Moses say God's people should do (see verses 1,13-14)?

_____

_____

_____

_____

What do you hear the Lord calling you to do today as you continue to yield your heart fully to Him?

_____

_____

_____

_____

Lord Jesus, thank You for dying for my sins and sending Your Holy Spirit so I can live a life of obedience. I look forward to following You today as You strengthen my devotion in seeking You. Amen.

Day 5

NEVER UNPROTECTED

Gracious Lord, thank You for another day to learn about Your power, love and judgment. Teach me to protect my heart from turning away from You.

Hank Williams recorded 35 singles that made it to the top of the Billboard Country and Western Best charts. Eleven of those singles made it to #1. In many ways, Williams defined country music for a generation. However, what many people don't realize is that Williams died of a heart attack when he was only 29. Despite warnings from family and friends, he chose to live a life that led to his early death.

Unfortunately, many people today also ignore the warning to guard their hearts and continue down a path of destruction until it's too late. In the Bible one such man who did this was King Solomon. As he grew older, Solomon left his heart unguarded against his father's warning (see

1 Kings 2:3), and he allowed other loves to turn him away from seeking the Lord. Read 1 Kings 3:7-15. What did Solomon ask God to give him (see verses 7-9)?

_____

_____

_____

_____

God was pleased by Solomon's request and promised to give him much more than he wanted. However, what was the condition that Solomon had to fulfill in order to experience a long and healthy life (see verse 14)?

_____

_____

_____

_____

Solomon began his walk with the Lord in obedience, doing everything God required, and he became known as one of the wisest kings in the world. At the dedication of the Temple, the Lord once again set out a promise and warning for Solomon. Read 1 Kings 9:1-9. What promise did the Lord make to him, and what warning did He give?

_____

_____

_____

_____

Read 1 Kings 11:1-13. What turned Solomon's heart away from the Lord (see verses 1-8)?

_____

_____

_____

_____

As a result of Solomon's disobedience, what did God plan to do (see verses 9-13)?

_____

_____

_____

_____

_____

According to Psalm 91:14-15, why will God protect us?

_____

_____

_____

_____

What can you do to actively participate in the spiritual protection of your heart?

_____

_____

_____

_____

> *Lord, keep my heart open to You, for You want me to succeed. Help me protect my heart so that I will stay devoted to You and protected by You. Amen.*

Day 6 REFLECTION AND APPLICATION

Gracious Lord, I've done things that I am ashamed of, and I need Your forgiveness. Please heal my past and help me to move beyond the guilt I feel in my broken heart. Thank You, Lord. Amen.

Have you ever questioned God's desire and ability to forgive and heal your past so that your heart can be truly cleansed? Do you really think that you could do anything that God would not forgive if you asked

Him? Read 1 John 3:19-22. Although we might occasionally allow our hearts to condemn us, why can our hearts still rest in God's presence (see verse 20)?

_____

_____

_____

_____

_____

Why do you think people allow their hearts to overrule what God wants for them?

_____

_____

_____

_____

_____

How can we have hearts that do not condemn us (see verses 21-22)?

_____

_____

_____

_____

When we allow Jesus to rule and take hold in our hearts, He actively helps us to follow His teachings. Jesus did not die so that we could be forgiven but still live in guilt. He died so that we might live in freedom. As you spend some quiet time with God today, ask Him to show you any areas of your life where there are some hidden feelings of guilt. Talk to Him about anything in your past that you feel holds you back from feeling His forgiveness, mercy and love.

Lord Jesus, thank You for being greater than my heart that sometimes condemns me. I receive Your love and forgiveness. Use my life to Your glory. Amen.

REFLECTION AND APPLICATION

*My heart is devoted to You, O Lord, and I seek Your presence in my life. I
want You to be the heart of my life. Because You heal, protect and preserve, I
know that I can live a life of health and hope. Amen.*

God has made it clear that He loves us, but sometimes we think that we
can make Him love us more or get more of His attention by *doing* more
and more. But nothing we have done will make God love us less, and
nothing we will do will make God love us more. We simply have to remain in His love.

In John 15:9-11, Jesus says, "As the Father has loved me, so have I
loved you. Now remain in my love. If you obey my commands, you will
remain in my love, just as I have obeyed my Father's commands and remain in his love. I have told you this so that my joy may be in you and
that your joy may be complete." God wants our lives to be full of joy!
And what does He ask of us? Our obedience. When our hearts are in the
right condition—when we believe that God loves us and when we show
that we love God—we will see God working in us, in our immediate sur-
roundings, and in the world.

So how's your heart? During the past week, you have had a chance
to do some good heart work. Now it's time for a heart checkup. Give a
general evaluation of the state of your heart using the following scale:

1	2	3	4	5	6	7	8	9	10
Ready to explode				Needs work		Pretty good			Pure

Now write down a few specific ways that you can care for your heart in
each of the four areas of your life.

Physical

_____

_____

_____

Mental

_____

_____

_____

_____

Emotional

_____

_____

_____

_____

Spiritual

_____

_____

_____

_____

Keep in mind Paul's words in Galatians 5:6: "The only thing that counts is faith expressing itself through love."

Lord of my heart, I give You my will, my thoughts and my actions. Shape my spirit to conform to Your great love. I want to show the world that You are working through me, and I want the world to see You working in the world. I love You. Amen.

Group Prayer Requests

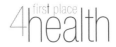

Today's Date: _____

Name	Request

Results

_____

_____

_____

_____

_____

time to
celebrate!

To help shape your brief victory celebration testimony, work through the following questions in your prayer journal:

Day One: List some of the benefits you have gained by allowing the Lord to transform your life through this 12-week First Place 4 Health session. Be sure to list benefits you have received in the physical, mental, emotional and spiritual realms of your being.

Day Two: In what ways have you most significantly changed *mentally*? Have you seen a shift in the ways you think about yourself, food, your relationships or God? How has Scripture memory been a part of these shifts?

Day Three: In what ways have you most significantly changed *emotionally*? Have you begun to identify how your feelings influence your relationship to food and exercise? What are you doing to stay aware of your emotions, both positive and negative?

Day Four: In what ways have you most significantly changed *spiritually*? How has your relationship with God deepened? How has drawing closer to Him made a difference in the other three areas of your life?

Day Five: In what ways have you most significantly changed *physically*? Have you met or exceeded your weight/measurement goals? How has your health improved the past 12 weeks?

Day Six: Was there one person in your First Place 4 Health group who was particularly encouraging to you? How did their kindness make a difference in your First Place 4 Health journey?

Day Seven: Summarize the previous six questions into a one-page testimony, or "faith story," to share at your group's victory celebration.

May our gracious Lord bless and keep you as you continue to keep Him first in all things!

Motivated to Wellness
leader discussion guide

For in-depth information, guidance and helpful tips about leading a successful First Place 4 Health group, spend time studying the *First Place 4 Health Leader's Guide*. In it, you will find valuable answers to most of your questions, as well as personal insights from many First Place 4 Health group leaders.

For the group meetings in this session, be sure to read and consider each week's discussion topics several days before the meeting—some questions and activities require supplies and/or planning to complete. Also, if you are leading a large group, plan to break into smaller groups for discussion and then come together as a large group to share your answers and responses. Make sure to appoint a capable leader for each small group so that discussions stay focused and on track (and be sure each group records their answers!).

week one: welcome to *Motivated to Wellness*

During this first week, welcome the members to your group, provide a brief overview of the First Place 4 Health program, explain what is expected of the participants at each of the weekly meetings, and collect the Member Surveys. (See the *First Place 4 Health Leader's Guide* for a detailed outline of how to conduct the first week's meeting.)

week two: finding hope to run the race

Prior to the meeting, ask someone in the group who journals regularly to be ready to talk about the benefits of keeping a journal. Open the session with prayer, using the words from Psalm 40:4 to begin your prayer.

Recite Psalm 40:4 and have the group read aloud verses 1-4. Ask several people to share what verse 4 means to them personally in general.

On a whiteboard, write the words "Running Theology." Have a volunteer read Hebrews 12:1-4. Write "Run Free" (see Day 1). As a group, develop a list of common activities and/or thoughts that entangle people and hinder them from running free in their walk with Christ and their desire to live a healthy life.

Write "Run with Perseverance" (see Day 2). Break into small groups and ask each group to develop three creative ways a person can keep his or her eyes on Jesus when difficulties are encountered.

Write "Never Run Alone" (see Day 3). Discuss how important having a support system is. Ask for specific ways members can offer support to each other. Ask each member to describe someone who has given him or her hope and to explain what it is about this person that is so inspiring.

Write "Run Your Own Race" (see Day 4). Give each member a magazine and ask them each to find one example of an enticement to follow some standard that our culture values (appearance, financial status, address, and so forth). Discuss the conflict we feel between wanting to live the way the world suggests and wanting to live the way God says is best.

Write "Run Focused" (see Day 5). Ask the group to suggest specific ways to keep our eyes focused on Jesus (prayer, Bible study, keeping a journal, and so forth). End the meeting with a prayer, encouraging each person to make a commitment to trust God and focus on Jesus.

week three: avoiding the lies and walking in the light

Begin this session with prayer, using the words of Psalm 89:15 to begin your prayer. Invite each group member to speak words of praise to God by completing this sentence: "Lord, I praise You because . . ." Together, have the group recite Psalm 89:15.

Invite the group to perform a dramatic reading of Jesus healing the blind man from John 9 (see Day 1). Invite volunteers to read the parts of Jesus, the blind man, the blind man's parents, the disciples, the Pharisees, and one person to speak for the neighbors. Encourage them to be very expressive. Afterward, discuss why the Pharisees were upset about the healing (it was the Sabbath; they didn't believe the man was actually born blind; a sinner couldn't have healed the man, so who was Jesus really?); and discuss why the Pharisees were guilty of being blind (they were shown the truth but still they refused to believe).

Have the members form small groups, and give them a few minutes to brainstorm the many lies our culture tells us that steal our identity, kill our joy or destroy our relationship with God (see Day 2). Bring the group back together and list the lies on a whiteboard. After the group identifies three or four common lies, encourage the group to find Scripture passages that speak directly to those lies.

Make sure that everyone in the group understands the significance of John 3:16 and the fact that God's love is a gift, not something we can earn (see Day 3). With the group, brainstorm and list on a whiteboard the false gods (fame, money, and so forth) that most of our society worships (see Day 4). Invite the group to talk about what parts of their commitment to First Place 4 Health will keep them from being split between following God's best for their lives and believing the lies.

Ask a volunteer to read 1 Corinthians 2:16 (see Day 6). Invite the group to share ways that can be used to further develop the mind of Christ in each of us. After sharing, ask the group to discuss what they can do each day to show that they have the mind of Christ. Close in prayer, inviting each person to again praise God.

week four: embracing a new way of thinking

Begin this session with a prayer that begins with the following: "Lord, each day we have moments when we feel as if we are in a desert. Thank You that in those times You want to do a new thing." Have the group recite Isaiah 43:19 together.

Have each member write down on an index card one experience from the past that holds him or her back from experiencing God's work today (see Day 1). Invite those who are comfortable to share their experiences. Then remind the group members that the Lord calls them to forget the past and to watch for His new work. As a symbolic act, have each person rip the card into pieces and drop the pieces into a trash can.

Invite a volunteer to read aloud Psalm 1, and encourage the group to talk about ways to delight in God's Word (see Day 2). Make a list on a whiteboard of ways to meditate on God's Word throughout the day.

Write 2 Corinthians 5:17 on a whiteboard. Under the verse write "Old Habits" and "New Habits," making two columns. Ask the group to list old habits that have been changing and new habits that are beginning to take hold in their lives. Discuss how being a new creation in Christ makes this change possible.

Ask the group to list things that are true, noble, pure, lovely or admirable. Discuss why thinking about such things is so difficult.

Draw a cross on the whiteboard. Ask the group to tell how our horizontal relationships (referring to the cross beam) can help us to live as Jesus calls us to live. Then encourage the group to consider their vertical relationship with God and how that can help them be successful in reaching their First Place 4 Health goals. Close in prayer asking the Lord to create a new way of thinking in each person.

week five: overcoming obstacles and training for success

Begin this session with a prayer that ends with Galatians 6:9-10: "Let us not become weary in doing good, for at the proper time we will reap a harvest if we do not give up. Therefore, as we have opportunity, let us do good to all people, especially to those who belong to the family of believers." As a group, recite Galatians 6:9 together.

On a whiteboard, write the words "Grow weary" and "Ready to Do Good," making two columns (see Day 1). Ask the group to identify words that describe the experience of growing weary and words that describe the experience of feeling ready to do good. Ask volunteers to share a time when they grew weary but kept going and ended up experiencing a feeling that is listed in the second column.

Have the group discuss ways to use their time more effectively and ways to increase the quality of time they spend in exercise, with family and in their quiet time (see Day 2). Also talk about why gaining hearts of wisdom is so important and what that wisdom will enable us to do.

Ask a volunteer to read aloud Ecclesiastes 4:9-12 (see Day 3). Have the members form two groups, and ask one group to discuss and write out the benefits of having a partner in a wellness plan, while the other group talks about and writes out the pitfalls of not having a partner. Ask for volunteers to share a personal experience that demonstrates a benefit or a pitfall.

Invite the members to share their experiences of crying out to the Lord and having their needs met (see Day 4). If you have time, read Psalm 118, asking each person to choose a phrase that he or she finds helpful and encouraging.

On a whiteboard, write "joyful in hope" centered at the top, "patient in affliction" in the left-hand corner, and "faithful in prayer" in the right-hand corner (see Day 5). Draw a line between them to make a triangle. Talk with the group about how these three patterns of life are connected, which is easiest to do and which is the most common in their experiences. End the session with a prayer asking the Lord to encourage the members of the group to continue on their fitness journeys.

week six: sustaining motivation from the Word of God

Begin the session with a brief prayer. Then turn off all the lights and light a votive candle in the middle of your meeting space. When you turn on the lights, ask the group to identify parts of the room still in the dark. Explain that we need God's light to touch every part of our lives. Ask the group to share why they may or may not want God to search them.

Discuss how Romans 12:3 would be helpful to both an overly proud person and a person with low self-esteem (see Day 2). Also talk about the ways both of them need to understand grace.

Have the group reflect on times when they were living the farthest from God's light, and remind them that at that time God loved them with extravagance. Ask for volunteers to share how the Lord brought the light of grace into their lives.

Invite a volunteer to tell what the two greatest commandments are and then discuss with the group why those particular commandments are the greatest ones. Also, ask group members to share the specific ways they thought of to show love to God with their hearts, souls, minds and strength. Discuss who our neighbors are (including First Place 4 Health members) and ways to show love to them.

Have the group reflect on God's promise that Jesus spoke in Matthew 11:28-30 (see Day 4). Discuss the benefits of being yoked with another person and the benefits of being yoked to Jesus. Ask the group to describe how they feel about being a temple, a dwelling place, for the Holy Spirit (see Day 5). Have volunteers describe how knowing this can motivate a person to improve their lifestyle and pursue a life of wellness.

Close the session with a prayer for the success of each member, and give thanks for the work God has already done. Then turn off the lights, light the candle you used at the beginning of the session, and have everyone recite Psalm 119:148 together.

week seven: living a life of worship

Have a bowl of fresh grapes and a bowl full of raisins on the table as the group members gather. You will refer to the grapes later in the study. Begin the session with prayer, and recite Psalm 105:4 as a group.

Have the group discuss why "living sacrifice" is not a contradiction in terms (see Day 1). Ask the group members to talk about why it might be difficult to stop conforming to the world and why our transformation is not instantaneous but takes time to accomplish.

Invite volunteers to explain why some people have trouble finding time to pray to God and spend time alone with Him (see Day 2).

Have a volunteer summarize the story of King David and Araunah in 1 Chronicles 21:14-26. Point out that King David brought judgment on Israel when he took a census, probably in order to show that he had powerful forces or to show that he had a large number of forces. Discuss why David didn't accept the free gift that Araunah offered. Ask volunteers to tell some ways that people today seek to please God without making any sort of sacrifice. Also ask the group how their experiences in First Place 4 Health work against taking the easy way out of getting healthy.

Write the word "sanctification" on a whiteboard (see Day 4). Explain that sanctification means being set apart for Christ; it means growing in grace to become more and more like Christ. Ask volunteers to tell why they do or do not feel holy and discuss why maintaining a relationship with Jesus is important to maintaining our holiness.

Turn the group's attention to the grapes and raisins and ask them to describe the difference between the two. Point out that grapes are plump and full, but when they're removed from the vines, they stop growing and begin to dry out, becoming raisins. Read John 15:5-6 and discuss what remaining in Christ means.

Point out that worshiping God in spirit and truth enhances the process of sanctification (see Day 5). Discuss what steps someone can take to develop a daily attitude of worshiping God in spirit and truth. On the whiteboard, list some ways the members came up with to worship God physically, mentally, emotionally and spiritually (see Day 6).

Close in prayer, giving thanks for the ways the Lord is working in each person's life.

week eight: taking time to rest

Open the study by asking everyone where they go when they need to escape and rest. After each person shares, say a prayer that includes thanks for the variety of places to rest that the Lord gives us. Ask the group to recite Luke 10:41-42 together.

Ask the group whether they identify more with Martha or Mary (see Day 1) and which woman society would favor. Ask a volunteer to explain why Mary's choice was better and what Jesus meant when He said, "It will not be taken away from her."

Briefly review the story of the birds and flowers told in Matthew 6:25-34 (see Day 2). Ask for ideas about what worrying *does* do to us (raises blood pressure, prevents restful sleep, shortens tempers). Then have a volunteer read 1 Peter 5:7.

Mention again the places of rest the group described at the beginning of the session. Ask if these places could also become places to experience the Sabbath. Discuss the reasons people give for not following God's command to keep the Sabbath holy.

Ask a volunteer to read aloud Psalm 127:1-2 (see Day 4). Discuss how these verses reinforce the need for sleep and rest and how they reinforce the idea of casting our anxieties on the Lord.

Talk about the ways that the Sabbath would be dishonored according to Isaiah 58:13 (see Day 5). Then ask for other ways in which the Sabbath can be dishonored. Have volunteers share how they usually spend the Sabbath and whether they are honoring or dishonoring God. Invite the group to share reasons why rest is necessary in all areas of life.

Close with prayer, encouraging the group members to rest in the Lord and to honor His Sabbath.

week nine: finding strength for a lifetime

Begin the session with a prayer. Have a variety of weights and resistance bands in the center of the table as the group members arrive. Ask everyone to suggest a benefit of weight training. Say a prayer that focuses on gaining strength as we hope in the Lord.

Have the members form three groups, and assign each group either Caleb, Joshua or Samson (see Days 1, 2 and 3). Give the small groups time to answer the following questions, and then bring the groups back together to share their answers.

Caleb: What two situations did Caleb face that tested his core strength? What words did Caleb use to show his dependence on the Lord? What were the results of Caleb's actions? What do you learn from Caleb's life that encourages your core confidence in the Lord?

Joshua: What did Joshua face that tested his core strength? What words did the Lord give Joshua to strengthen his core? What was the result of Joshua's putting God's Word into practice? What do you learn from Joshua's life that encourages your core confidence in the Lord?

Samson: What situation did Samson face at the end of his life that tested his core strength? What prayer did Samson pray to show his dependence on the Lord? What was the result of Samson's action? What do you learn from Samson's life that can help you build your strength in the Lord?

Have a volunteer read Psalm 31:9-18 (see Day 4). Ask the group to tell how David felt (verses 9-13) and on what he depended (verses 14-18). Ask the group to tell how a person can demonstrate that he or she trusts in God.

Ask the group members if there are areas in their lives they feel the Lord has healed or is in the process of healing as a result of their participation in the First Place 4 Health program. Ask if there are places where they still feel paralyzed. Take time to pray specifically for those who need and want healing.

Invite members to share how worry can sap a person's strength. Have a few volunteers share their examples of people who have encouraged their Christian walks, and on a whiteboard, write a list of the action steps the members of the group will take to encourage someone else's walk (see Day 7).

As you close the meeting, pray for each member to build his or her physical core strength and spiritual core strength in the Lord.

week ten: stretching for the Lord

Begin the session with a prayer. On a whiteboard, write the words "I can't" and "I can because God can" (see Day 1). Ask the group to share things in their lives that they didn't think they could do before they joined the First Place 4 Health program, and write their responses under "I can't." Under "I can because God can," write the answers the members give to explain how God has helped them to stretch and make progress toward their goals.

Discuss what sharing in the fellowship of Christ's suffering means (see Philippians 3:10) and how a person can be victorious, even though he or she is suffering. Ask volunteers to briefly describe a difficult situation they experienced that turned into a time of growth and change and restoration in their walk with Christ. Discuss how fear can make a person unbendable and afraid of change, even if the change is a good one.

Invite one person to briefly review the story of the man with the shriveled hand recorded in Matthew 12:9-14. Discuss the courage it took for the man to listen to Jesus and the faith the man had that he would be healed if he did what Jesus said to do. Then talk about the courage it takes for us to stretch beyond our lives and reach out to Jesus to bring us healing.

Ask a volunteer to briefly recap Peter's vision, how he initially reacted to God's instructions and what he eventually ended up accomplishing (see Day 5). Then have another volunteer recap what happened to the plans of Paul and his companions, recorded in Acts 16:6-10.

Ahead of time, search the Internet and print out pictures of Daniel Browning Smith (the Rubberboy) and the Golden Gate Bridge (see Days 6 and 7). Show the pictures and have volunteers share the areas of their walks with Christ that need to be more flexible and areas that need a stronger foundation.

As you end the study, pray for each member of the group to allow the Lord to continue to stretch and grow them in tremendous ways over the next week.

week eleven: caring for your heart

Begin the session with prayer. Have the group recite the memory verse (1 Chronicles 22:19) together. Then, on a whiteboard, list the priorities that people often hold higher than the Lord (see Day 1). Discuss how a person can keep God as the top priority while trying to meet the demands and expectations of life.

Draw a yield sign on the whiteboard (see Day 2). Discuss the positive and negative aspects of yielding to someone or something. Ask for ideas about how a person can remind himself or herself that he or she has committed to yield to God.

Discuss how keeping Scripture in our hearts builds a healthy heart, how prayer impacts the health of our heart, and what we need to prevent from entering our heart to keep things going strong. Ask each member to share how he or she is motivated: by the possibility of blessing or by the avoidance of pain (see Day 4). Ask the group to share their responses to the blessings and curses recorded in Deuteronomy 28.

On a whiteboard, write the words "Lessons from Solomon" (see Day 5). Have the group identify four to six lessons or principles that Solomon's life reveals about how a person can protect his or her heart.

A clean heart begins with forgiveness (see Day 6). Encourage the group to confess to God situations that are preventing them from experiencing the full love of Christ. Remind the group members that God promises to forgive those who ask, and He will heal them; and the Holy Spirit will bring hope into their lives.

At the close of the session, pray for cleansing and protection of each person's heart.

week twelve: time to celebrate!

Even though most of your meeting this week will be a victory celebration, take some time at the beginning of the meeting to talk about how much God loves each person in the group and how each of us is called to love our brothers and sisters in Christ. (See "Planning a Victory Celebration" in the *First Place 4 Health Leader's Guide* for ideas about throwing a successful celebration for your group.)

For the rest of the study time, allow each member to tell his or her *Motivated to Wellness* story. Give members an equal opportunity to share the goals they set for themselves at the beginning of the session and talk about the challenges and good things God has done for them throughout the process. Don't allow the more talkative group members to monopolize all the time. Even the quiet members need an opportunity to share their stories and successes! Even those who have not met their goals have still been part of the journey, so allow them to share and talk about why they did not succeed.

Making a commitment to continue in First Place 4 Health is an important part of victory. Be sure to talk about your group's future plans, and make each person feel welcome to continue to journey with you. End the study by inviting the group to proclaim together Hebrews 12:1-3.

First Place 4 Health menu plans

Each menu plan is based on approximately 1,400 to 1,500 calories per day. All recipe and menu exchanges were determined using the Master-Cook software, a program that accesses a database containing more than 6,000 food items prepared using the United States Department of Agriculture (USDA) publications and information from food manufacturers. As with any nutritional program, MasterCook calculates the nutritional values of the recipes based on ingredients. Nutrition may vary due to how the food is prepared, where the food comes from, soil content, season, ripeness, processing and method of preparation. For these reasons, please use the recipes and menu plans as approximate guides. Consult a physician and/or a registered dietitian before starting a weight-loss program.

For those who need more calories, add the following to the 1,400-calorie plan:

- 1,800 calories: 2 ounce equivalent of meat, 3 ounce equivalent of bread, ½ cup vegetable serving, 1 tsp. fat

- 2,000 calories: 2 ounce equivalent of meat, 4 ounce equivalent of bread, ½ cup vegetable serving, 3 tsp. fat

- 2,200 calories: 2 ounce equivalent of meat, 5 ounce equivalent of bread, ½ cup vegetable serving, ½ cup fruit serving, 5 tsp. fat

- 2,400 calories: 2 ounce equivalent of meat, 6 ounce equivalent of bread, 1 cup vegetable serving, ½ cup fruit serving, 6 tsp. fat

First Week Grocery List

Produce
- [ ] avocado
- [ ] bell peppers
- [ ] bibb lettuce
- [ ] blueberries
- [ ] carrots
- [ ] celery
- [ ] cilantro
- [ ] coleslaw mix
- [ ] garlic cloves
- [ ] golden raisins
- [ ] green bell peppers
- [ ] green onions
- [ ] honeydew melon
- [ ] jalapeño peppers
- [ ] limes
- [ ] mushrooms
- [ ] onions
- [ ] oranges
- [ ] parsley
- [ ] peaches
- [ ] raisins
- [ ] red apples
- [ ] red bell peppers
- [ ] romaine lettuce
- [ ] tomatoes
- [ ] Vidalia onion
- [ ] white onions
- [ ] yellow onion
- [ ] zucchini

Baking/Cooking Products
- [ ] baking powder
- [ ] brown sugar
- [ ] canola or vegetable oil
- [ ] chicken or vegetable bouillon cubes
- [ ] cornbread mix
- [ ] cornbread stuffing mix, herb-seasoned
- [ ] cornstarch
- [ ] flour
- [ ] nonstick cooking spray
- [ ] olive oil

Spices
- [ ] basil
- [ ] bay leaf
- [ ] black pepper
- [ ] cayenne pepper
- [ ] chili powder
- [ ] cinnamon
- [ ] Creole seasoning
- [ ] cumin
- [ ] Goya Adobo seasoning (or seasoned salt)
- [ ] Italian seasoning
- [ ] nutmeg
- [ ] oregano
- [ ] paprika
- [ ] poultry seasoning
- [ ] salt
- [ ] seasoned salt
- [ ] thyme
- [ ] white pepper

Nuts/Seeds
- [ ] walnuts

Condiments, Spreads and Sauces
- [ ] all-fruit spread
- [ ] applesauce, unsweetened
- [ ] Italian dressing, fat-free
- [ ] ketchup

- ❑ lime juice
- ❑ maple syrup, sugar-free
- ❑ mayonnaise, light
- ❑ mustard
- ❑ Parmesan cheese
- ❑ Pickapeppa sauce
- ❑ salsa
- ❑ Worcestershire sauce

Breads, Cereals and Pasta
- ❑ bagel
- ❑ Italian breadcrumbs
- ❑ bread, whole-wheat
- ❑ corn tortillas
- ❑ flour tortillas, fat-free
- ❑ Grape Nuts® cereal
- ❑ oatmeal
- ❑ pancakes, low-fat
- ❑ rice
- ❑ sourdough bread
- ❑ spaghetti
- ❑ tostada shells
- ❑ tube or macaroni pasta
- ❑ wheat flakes
- ❑ wheat germ

Canned/Frozen Foods
- ❑ beef broth, low-salt
- ❑ black beans
- ❑ broccoli
- ❑ cannelloni beans
- ❑ chicken or vegetable broth
- ❑ corn
- ❑ cream of chicken soup, reduced-fat
- ❑ garlic, minced
- ❑ green chiles
- ❑ Mandarin oranges
- ❑ Mexican corn, with red and green peppers

- ❑ pinto beans
- ❑ red kidney beans, lower-sodium
- ❑ spinach
- ❑ tomato paste
- ❑ tomato sauce, lower-sodium
- ❑ tomatoes, diced
- ❑ tomatoes, crushed
- ❑ tomatoes, diced with green chiles
- ❑ tomatoes, lower-sodium

Dairy Products
- ❑ blue cheese
- ❑ butter
- ❑ cottage cheese, 2%
- ❑ cream cheese, fat-free
- ❑ lemon yogurt, fat-free
- ❑ margarine, light
- ❑ margarine, regular
- ❑ milk, nonfat
- ❑ Monterey Jack cheese
- ❑ sour cream, low-fat
- ❑ Velveeta Light®
- ❑ yogurt, nonfat

Juices
- ❑ orange juice, calcium fortified

Meat and Poultry
- ❑ chicken breasts, skinless and boneless
- ❑ eggs
- ❑ flank steak
- ❑ ground beef, lean
- ❑ pancetta ham
- ❑ pork tenderloin
- ❑ rotisserie chicken breast

First Week Meals and Recipes

DAY 1

Breakfast

2 slices sourdough bread, toasted and topped with 1 tsp. light margarine

¾ cup blueberries
1 cup nonfat milk

Nutritional Information: 304 calories; 4g fat; 13g protein; 53g carbohydrate; 4g dietary fiber; 4mg cholesterol; 483mg sodium.

Lunch

Broccoli Cheese Soup

1 cup carrots, finely chopped
1 cup celery, finely chopped
1 cup green onions, finely chopped
1 (10-oz.) box frozen, chopped broccoli
1 medium white onion, chopped
2 cups water
4 tbsp. light margarine
1 cup flour

4 cups nonfat milk
4 cups fat-free, lower-sodium chicken broth (or vegetable broth)
1 lb. Velveeta Light® processed cheese, cut in small cubes
1 tsp. salt
1 tsp. black pepper
¼ tsp. cayenne pepper (optional)
1 tbsp. prepared mustard

In medium saucepan, bring water, broccoli, carrots, celery, onions and green onions to a boil. Cover pan and remove from heat. Set aside. In large stock pot, melt margarine over low heat. Stir in flour quickly to form a paste. When blended, remove from heat and mash out as many lumps as possible. Return pot to medium heat. Add milk and broth to margarine/flour mixture using a wire whisk to get out extra lumps of flour. When well blended, add cheese, salt, pepper and cayenne; stir until cheese melts. Add mustard and boiled vegetables, including water; stir well and bring to boil. Serve immediately. Serves 16.

Nutritional Information: 184 calories; 7g fat; 13g protein; 17g carbohydrate; 1g dietary fiber; 19mg cholesterol; 990mg sodium.

Dinner

Beef and Chicken Fajita with Pinto Beans

Marinade:

¼ cup olive oil	1 tsp. salt
1 tsp. grated lime rind	½ tsp. dried oregano
2½ tbsp. fresh lime juice	½ tsp. black pepper
2 tbsp. Worcestershire sauce	2 garlic cloves, minced
1½ tsp. ground cumin	1 (14¼-oz.) can low-salt beef broth

Fajitas:

1 (1-lb.) flank steak	1 large Vidalia or other sweet onion,
1 lb. chicken breast, skinless, boneless	cut into 16 wedges
2 red bell peppers, each cut into	16 (6-inch) fat-free flour tortillas
12 wedges	1 cup bottled salsa
2 green bell peppers, each cut into	¼ cup low-fat sour cream
12 wedges	½ cup chopped fresh cilantro
cilantro, fresh	nonstick cooking spray

To prepare marinade, combine olive oil, lime rind, fresh lime juice, Worcestershire sauce, cumin, salt, oregano, black pepper, garlic cloves and beef broth in a large bowl and set aside. To prepare fajitas, trim fat from steak. Score a diamond pattern on both sides of the steak. Combine 1½ cups marinade, steak and chicken in a large zip-top plastic bag. Seal and marinate in refrigerator 4 hours or overnight, turning occasionally. Combine remaining marinade, bell peppers and onion in a zip-top plastic bag. Seal and marinate in refrigerator for 4 hours or overnight, turning occasionally.

Prepare grill. Remove steak and chicken from bag; discard marinade. Remove vegetables from bag; reserve marinade. Place reserved marinade in a small saucepan; set aside. Place steak, chicken, and vegetables on grill rack coated with cooking spray; cook 8 minutes on each side or until desired degree of doneness. Wrap tortillas tightly in foil; place tortilla packet on grill rack the last 2 minutes of grilling time. Bring reserved marinade to a boil. Cut steak and chicken diagonally across the grain into thin slices. Place the steak, chicken, and vegetables on a serving platter; drizzle with reserved marinade. Arrange about 1 ounce steak, about 1 ounce chicken, 3 bell pepper wedges and 1 onion wedge in a tortilla; top with 1 tablespoon salsa, about 1 teaspoon sour cream and ½ tablespoon cilantro. Fold sides of tortilla over filling. Garnish with cilantro sprigs, if desired. Serve with *Pinto Beans a la Juan* (see recipe below). Serves 8.

Nutritional Information: 407 calories; 14.2g fat; 31.1g protein; 40.6g carbohydrate; 5.3g dietary fiber; 64mg cholesterol; 841mg sodium.

Pinto Beans a la Juan

2 lbs. pinto beans, rinsed well
10 quarts water
6 whole garlic cloves
2 large onions, coarsely chopped
(used separately)
1 tbsp. chili powder
1 tbsp. Creole seasoning
1 tbsp. cumin

1 tbsp. Goya Adobo Seasoning
(or seasoned salt)
1 tsp. salt
2 medium bell peppers, coarsely
chopped
4 tomatoes, coarsely chopped
1 bunch cilantro, rinsed and tied
together

In large pot, bring water, beans, 1 chopped onion, garlic and spices to a boil. Reduce heat and boil gently 1½ hours. Taste for seasoning, and add more seasonings if desired. Continue boiling gently about 3 hours more or until beans start getting soft. Add peppers, tomatoes, remaining onion and cilantro and cook 30 minutes more. Remove cilantro and discard before serving. Serves 16.

Nutritional Information: 221 calories; 1g fat; 13g protein; 41g carbohydrate; 15g dietary fiber; 0mg cholesterol; 217mg sodium.

DAY 2

Breakfast

1 cup oatmeal with ¼ tsp. light margarine, dash nutmeg, dash cinnamon, 1 cup nonfat milk and 2 tbsp. raisins

Nutritional Information: 284 calories; 3g fat; 15g protein; 50g carbohydrate; 5g dietary fiber; 4mg cholesterol; 517mg sodium.

Lunch

Vegetable Brunch Casserole and Creamy Fruit Salad

1 medium zucchini, diced
1 medium onion, chopped
8 oz. sliced mushrooms

¼ cup butter
½ cup flour
1 tsp. baking powder

½ tsp. salt
10 eggs, lightly beaten
2 cups (16 oz.) 2% cottage cheese
1 (3-oz.) can chopped green chilies

4 cups (16 oz.) shredded Monterey
  Jack Cheese
nonstick cooking spray

In a large skillet, sauté the zucchini, onion and mushrooms in butter until tender. Stir in the flour, baking powder and salt until blended. In a large bowl, combine eggs and cottage cheese. Stir in vegetables, green chilies and Monterey jack cheese. Set oven to 350° F. Spray a 13″ x 9″ pan with nonstick cooking spray. Pour mixture into pan and bake uncovered for 35 to 45 minutes or until set and golden brown on top. Serve with *Creamy Fruit Salad* (see recipe below). Serves 12.

Nutritional Information: 302 calories; 20g fat; 21g protein; 9g carbohydrate; 1g dietary fiber; 224mg cholesterol; 584mg sodium.

Creamy Fruit Salad

Dressing:
1 (6 oz.) fat-free lemon yogurt
1 tbsp. light mayonnaise

2 tbsp. orange juice

Salad:
2 large unpeeled red apples, cubed
  (about 3 cups)
15 oz. can of Mandarin oranges,
  drained

2 tbsp. golden raisins
2 tbsp. chopped walnuts
8 leaves bibb lettuce

In small bowl, mix dressing ingredients until well blended. In medium bowl, mix apples, oranges, raisins and walnuts. Pour dressing over fruit and toss gently to coat. Divide lettuce onto serving plates and top with fruit salad. Serves 8.

Nutritional Information: 82 calories; 2g fat; 1g protein; 18g carbohydrate; 2g dietary fiber; 1mg cholesterol; 13mg sodium.

Dinner

Spinach-topped Chicken

12 boneless, skinless chicken breasts
  (about 3½ lbs.)
3 egg whites
¾ cup Italian breadcrumbs
¼ cup grated Parmesan cheese
1 tsp. salt
1 tsp. black pepper

½ cup green onions, sliced
1 tbsp. minced garlic
4 oz. pancetta ham diced (or use
  chopped fresh mushroom for
  less calories)
2 tbsp. butter
2 tbsp. flour

1 10-oz. package frozen chopped spinach, thawed and well drained

1 cup nonfat milk

Preheat oven to 350° F. Slightly beat egg whites in small bowl; set aside. Combine breadcrumbs, cheese, salt and pepper in shallow dish. Dip chicken breasts in egg whites; roll in breadcrumb mixture and arrange in 9" x 13" baking dish. Save remaining crumbs. In a saucepan, cook green onions and garlic in butter until tender. Stir in flour. Stir in milk all at once. Cook and stir until thickened and bubbly. Cook and stir one minute more. Stir in spinach and ham (or mushrooms). Spoon spinach mixture over chicken; sprinkle with remaining crumb mixture. Bake uncovered 40 to 45 minutes or until done. Serves 12.

Nutritional Information: 211 calories; 5g fat; 31g protein; 8g carbohydrate; 1g dietary fiber; 79mg cholesterol; 391mg sodium.

Serve with wild rice and fresh steamed vegetables.

DAY 3

Breakfast

1 cup wheat flakes cereal
1 cup nonfat milk

1 medium peach, sliced

Nutritional Information: 253 calories; 3g fat; 18g protein; 60g carbohydrate; 27g dietary fiber; 4mg cholesterol; 127mg sodium.

Lunch

Chicken and Guacamole Tostadas

1 ripe avocado, peeled
1 cup plus 2 tbsp. finely chopped tomato, divided
3 tbsp. minced fresh onion, divided
3 tbsp. fresh lime juice, divided
½ tsp. salt, divided
1 small garlic clove, minced

1 tbsp. chopped fresh cilantro
1 tbsp. minced, seeded jalapeño pepper
2 cups shredded skinless, boneless rotisserie chicken breast
¼ tsp. smoked paprika
8 (6-inch) corn tostada shells

Place avocado in a small bowl and mash with a fork. Stir in 2 tablespoons tomato, 1 tablespoon onion, 1 tablespoon lime juice, ¼ teaspoon salt and garlic. Make salsa by combining remaining 1 cup tomato, 2 tablespoons onion, 1 tablespoon lime juice, ¼ teaspoon salt, cilantro and jalapeño; toss well. Combine chicken, remaining 1 tablespoon lime juice and paprika; toss well to combine. Spread about 1 tablespoon guacamole over each tostada shell; top each with ¼ cup chicken mixture and about 2 tablespoons salsa. Serves 4.

Nutritional Information: 345 calories; 15.4g fat; 25.4g protein; 26.9g carbohydrate; 5.4g dietary fiber; 60mg cholesterol; 548mg sodium.

Serve with a fresh fruit salad.

Dinner
Cajun Meat Loaf

2 lbs. lean ground beef
¾ cup onions, finely chopped
¼ cup green onion tops, finely chopped
½ cup chopped celery, finely chopped
½ cup bell pepper, finely chopped
2 tsp. minced garlic
4 tbsp. Pickapeppa sauce (or your favorite steak sauce), divided

1 tbsp. Worcestershire sauce
1 cup ketchup, divided
½ cup nonfat milk
3 egg whites
1 cup Italian breadcrumbs
1 tsp. salt
½ tsp. cayenne pepper
1 tsp. black pepper
nonstick cooking spray

Preheat oven to 375° F. In small bowl, combine ½ cup ketchup and 1 tablespoon Pickapeppa sauce; stir well and set aside. In large bowl, combine ground beef, onions, celery, bell pepper, garlic, remaining Pickapeppa, Worcestershire sauce, ½ cup ketchup, milk, egg whites, breadcrumbs, salt, cayenne and black peppers; mix well. Spray large baking dish with nonstick cooking spray. Place meat mixture into pan and shape into a loaf. Bake uncovered 45 minutes. Remove loaf; spread with ketchup sauce and return to oven. Cook meat loaf 30 minutes more or until done. (*Note*: You can also make 10 mini loaves, but the cooking time will be less.) Serves 10.

Nutritional Information: 301 calories; 16g fat; 21g protein; 18g carbohydrate; 1g dietary fiber; 63mg cholesterol; 695mg sodium.

Serve with fresh squash and mashed potatoes.

DAY 4

Breakfast
Quick Bagel Breakfast

½ large bagel, toasted
2 tbsp. fat-free cream cheese

1 small orange
1 cup nonfat milk

Nutritional Information: 335 calories; 6g fat; 17g protein; 53g carbohydrate; 4g dietary fiber; 20mg cholesterol; 523mg sodium.

Lunch
Easy Chef Salad with Chicken

10 cups chopped romaine lettuce
1 cup shredded skinless, boneless
  rotisserie chicken breast
½ cup sweet onion, thinly sliced

⅓ cup carrot, grated
1 avocado, seeded, peeled and sliced
3 tbsp. crumbled blue cheese
½ cup fat-free Italian dressing

Arrange 2½ cups lettuce on each of 4 plates. Top lettuce evenly with chicken, onion, carrot, avocado and blue cheese. Drizzle each serving with 2 tablespoons fat-free dressing; serve immediately. Serves 4.

Nutritional Information: 367 calories; 28.2g fat 18.5g protein; 12.6g carbohydrate; 4.6g dietary fiber; 43mg cholesterol; 451mg sodium.

Dinner

Spice-rubbed Pork Tenderloin

1 clove garlic, minced
1 tsp. seasoned salt
1 tsp. white pepper and 1 tsp. black pepper
1 tsp. Italian seasoning

1 lb. pork tenderloin
1 tbsp. olive oil
cornstarch
nonstick cooking spray

Mix garlic and all seasonings in a small bowl. Rub mixture over tenderloin and wrap in plastic. Refrigerate for at least 4 hours. Heat olive oil in large skillet over medium-high heat and brown pork on all sides (about 7 minutes). Place pork in a 13" x 9" x 2" pan that has been sprayed with nonstick cooking spray. Add enough water to pan to come to bottom edge of pork (about a half inch). Cover with foil and bake at 350° F for 45 to 50 minutes or until a thermometer reaches 160° F. Pour the drippings in a pan and mix with a little cornstarch mixed with water to make the gravy; season gravy with salt and pepper. Serves 4.

Nutritional Information: 261 calories; 12.7g fat; 33.5g protein; 0.8g carbohydrate; 3g dietary fiber; 89mg cholesterol; 644mg sodium.

Serve with small tossed salad, steamed asparagus and a dinner roll.

DAY 5

Breakfast
French Toast

2 slices whole-wheat bread
1 egg, beaten

1 tbsp. light or 1 tsp. regular
  margarine

2 tbsp. sugar-free maple syrup,
  if desired
1 cup nonfat milk

½ cup unsweetened applesauce with
  dash of cinnamon
nonstick cooking spray

Dip 2 slices of bread in beaten egg. Brown on both sides in pan sprayed with nonstick cooking spray. Serve with margarine and sugar-free maple syrup (if desired) and unsweetened applesauce. Serves 1.

Nutritional Information: 395 calories; 13g fat; 19g protein; 51g carbohydrate; 3g dietary fiber; 217mg cholesterol; 606mg sodium.

....

Lunch
Mexican Chicken Casserole

10 oz. boneless, skinless chicken
  breasts, cooked and diced
12 (6-inch) corn tortillas, torn or cut
  into pieces
2 (10.7-oz.) cans reduced-fat cream
  of chicken soup
1 bell pepper, chopped

1 (10-oz.) can diced tomatoes with
  green chiles
8 oz. Velveeta Light® processed
  cheese
1 onion, chopped
nonstick cooking spray

Preheat oven to 350° F. In medium saucepan, heat soup, tomatoes and cheese until cheese is melted. Sauté bell pepper and onion in nonstick skillet with ¼ cup of water or broth until tender. Stir into soup mixture; add chicken and tortillas. Pour into 13″ x 9″ x 2″ baking dish coated with cooking spray. Bake 30 minutes or until bubbly. Serve with *Black Bean and Rice Salad* (see recipe below). Serves 8.

Nutritional Information: 243 calories; 7g fat; 20g protein; 26g carbohydrate; 3g dietary fiber; 38mg cholesterol; 989mg sodium.

Black Bean and Rice Salad

1 (11-oz.) can kernel corn, drained
1 (15-oz.) can black beans, drained
1 cup cooked rice, cooled
1 (4-oz) can green chiles, chopped
½ cup green onions, chopped

½ cup celery, chopped
½ cup red bell pepper, chopped
2 tbsp. fresh cilantro (optional)
¼ to ½ cup salsa or fat-free Italian
  dressing

Mix all together and refrigerate at least 4 hours. Serve over chopped lettuce. Serves 10.

Nutritional Information: 80 calories; 1g fat; 4g protein; 15g carbohydrate; 3g dietary fiber; 0mg cholesterol; 168mg sodium.

Dinner

Spaghetti with Meat Sauce

1 cup chopped onion
1 lb. lean ground beef
2 cloves garlic, minced
1 (1-lb. 14-oz.) can crushed tomatoes
1 (1-lb.) can diced tomatoes
1 (6-oz.) can tomato paste
2 cups water

¼ cup snipped parsley
1 tbsp. brown sugar
1 tsp. salt
1½ tsp. dried oregano, crushed
¼ tsp. dried thyme, crushed
1 bay leaf
12 oz. spaghetti (cooked)

In Dutch oven, combine onion, beef and garlic; cook until meat is browned and onion is tender. Skim off excess fat and add tomatoes, tomato paste, water, parsley, brown sugar, salt, oregano, thyme and bay leaf. Simmer uncovered for 2 to 3 hours or until sauce is thick, stirring occasionally. If too thick, add a little more water. Remove bay leaf. Serve over hot spaghetti. Serves 6.

Nutritional Information: 355 calories; 3g fat; 13g protein; 36g carbohydrate; 5g dietary fiber; 21mg cholesterol; 927mg sodium.

Serve with a small dinner salad and a bread stick.

DAY 6

Breakfast

2 slices whole-wheat toast
2 tsp. all-fruit spread
1 cup nonfat plain yogurt

3 tbsp. wheat germ or 2 tbsp. Grape Nuts® cereal
6 oz. calcium-fortified orange juice

Nutritional Information: 434 calories; 5g fat; 22g protein; 80g carbohydrate; 8g dietary fiber; 3mg cholesterol; 433mg sodium.

Lunch

Minestrone Soup

2 tsp. olive oil
¼ cup onion, chopped
1 tsp. garlic, chopped
3 cups vegetable broth or water
1 cup diced carrots
1 (15½-oz.) can cannelloni beans or other white bean (drained)
¾ cup diced celery

1 (14½-oz.) can diced tomatoes, not drained
½ tsp. dried basil
¼ tsp. salt
¼ tsp. dried oregano
½ tsp. black pepper
¼ cup uncooked macaroni pasta
4 tsp. Parmesan cheese

Heat oil in a large stockpot over medium heat; add onion and garlic and sauté until lightly browned. Add broth, carrots, beans, celery, tomatoes and spices and bring to a boil. Cover, reduce heat to medium, and cook for 25 minutes. Add pasta and cook for 10 minutes. Ladle into bowls and top with cheese. Serving size is about 1½ cups. Serves 4.

Nutritional Information: 176 calories; 3g fat; 9g protein; 30g carbohydrate; 4g; dietary fiber; trace cholesterol; 699mg sodium.

Dinner

Grilled Burger and Texas-style Coleslaw

1 bag (16-oz.) coleslaw mix	3 tbsp. canola or vegetable oil
½ cup chopped fresh cilantro	3 tbsp. lime juice
2 cans (11 oz. each) Mexican corn with red and green peppers, drained	½ tsp salt
	¾ tsp ground cumin

In a large bowl, toss coleslaw mix, cilantro and corn. In container with tight lid, shake oil, lime juice, salt and cumin until well mixed. Pour over coleslaw mixture; toss. Cover; refrigerate 1 to 2 hours to blend flavors before serving. Serves 16.

Nutritional Information: 70 calories; 3g fat; 2g protein; 9g carbohydrate; 1g dietary fiber; 0mg cholesterol; 210mg sodium.

DAY 7

Breakfast

2 frozen low fat pancakes, heated	2-inch wedge honeydew melon
1 tbsp. sugar-free maple syrup	1 cup nonfat milk
1 tsp. light margarine	

Nutritional Information: 379 calories; 5g fat; 14g protein; 73g carbohydrate; 3g dietary fiber; 11mg cholesterol; 571mg sodium.

Lunch

Cornbread Dressing with Gravy

Cornbread Dressing:

2 (6-oz.) packets cornbread mix	1½ cups celery, chopped
2 whole eggs	9 cups water
1⅓ cups nonfat milk	9 chicken bouillon cubes (or vegetable)
1½ cups onion, chopped	
1 (8-oz.) package herb-seasoned cornbread stuffing mix	1 tbsp. poultry seasoning
	4 egg whites (or 2 eggs)

Make cornbread according to package directions, using the 2 whole eggs and nonfat milk. Let cool. (Can even be done the day ahead). Boil celery and onion in the water with the bouillon cubes over low heat for 3 to 5 minutes. Crumble cooked cornbread and combine with stuffing mix. Pour boiled vegetable mixture over bread mixture and add poultry seasoning. Pour into a large casserole dish. After mixture has cooled, stir in beaten egg whites. Bake at 375° F for 60 to 90 minutes or until crusty and brown on top. Serve with *Cornbread Dressing Gravy* (see recipe below). Serves 16.

Nutritional Information: 124 calories; 3g fat; 5g protein; 19g carbohydrate; 2g dietary fiber; 27mg cholesterol; 766mg sodium.

Cornbread Dressing Gravy:

3¾ cups water (divided)
4 chicken/vegetable bouillon cubes

2 tbsp. flour (or cornstarch)
salt and black pepper, to taste

In 2-quart saucepan, bring 3 cups water to boil and add bouillon cubes. In a pint jar with lid, combine ¾ cup water with flour; shake well. Slowly pour into boiling water, stirring constantly to prevent lumps. Simmer over low heat, stirring frequently until gravy consistency is reached. Add flour or water if needed to reach desired consistency. Add salt and pepper to taste. Serves 16.

Nutritional Information: 6 calories; trace fat; trace protein; 1g carbohydrate; trace dietary fiber; trace cholesterol; 188mg sodium.

....

Dinner

Texas Chili with Beans

8 oz. lean ground beef
1 cup onion, chopped
1 cup celery, chopped
½ cup green pepper, chopped
2 cloves garlic, minced
1 (15½-oz.) can lower-sodium red
  kidney beans, drained
¼ cup water

1 (14½-oz.) can lower-sodium
  tomatoes, cut up
1 (8-oz.) can lower-sodium
  tomato sauce
2 to 3 tsp. chili powder (to taste)
½ tsp. salt
½ tsp. dried basil, crushed
¼ tsp. black pepper

Cook ground beef, onion, celery, green pepper and garlic until meat is brown. Drain off fat. Stir in kidney beans, undrained tomatoes, tomato sauce, water, chili powder, salt, basil and pepper. Bring to boiling; reduce heat. Cover and simmer for 25 to 30 minutes or till the vegetables are tender. Serves 4.

Nutritional Information: 305 calories; 13g fat; 18g protein; 31g carbohydrate; 11g dietary fiber; 43mg cholesterol; 957mg sodium.

Second Week Grocery List

Produce
- [ ] bananas
- [ ] basil
- [ ] bell peppers
- [ ] broccoli
- [ ] cabbage
- [ ] cantaloupe
- [ ] carrots
- [ ] cauliflower
- [ ] celery
- [ ] chives
- [ ] cilantro
- [ ] fresh parsley
- [ ] garlic cloves
- [ ] grapefruit
- [ ] green onions
- [ ] jalapeño pepper
- [ ] limes
- [ ] mushrooms
- [ ] onions
- [ ] oranges
- [ ] parsley
- [ ] radishes
- [ ] red onions
- [ ] red bell pepper
- [ ] red potatoes
- [ ] romaine lettuce
- [ ] tomatoes
- [ ] yellow squash
- [ ] zucchini

Baking/Cooking Products
- [ ] breadcrumbs
- [ ] cornstarch
- [ ] dark brown sugar
- [ ] dark corn syrup
- [ ] flour, all-purpose
- [ ] light brown sugar
- [ ] nonstick cooking spray

- [ ] olive oil
- [ ] peanut oil
- [ ] piecrust, unbaked
- [ ] vanilla extract

Spices
- [ ] Allspice
- [ ] basil
- [ ] basil pesto
- [ ] bay leaf, dried
- [ ] black pepper
- [ ] black peppercorns
- [ ] chili powder
- [ ] cumin
- [ ] dill
- [ ] garlic powder
- [ ] Italian seasoning
- [ ] mustard
- [ ] onion powder
- [ ] oregano
- [ ] paprika
- [ ] parsley
- [ ] salt

Nuts/Seeds
- [ ] almonds, slivered
- [ ] peanuts, dry roasted, unsalted
- [ ] pecans
- [ ] pine nuts
- [ ] walnuts

Condiments, Spreads and Sauces
- [ ] chili sauce
- [ ] chocolate syrup
- [ ] peanut butter, creamy
- [ ] Dijon mustard
- [ ] Grand Marnier
- [ ] Honey
- [ ] Kitchen Bouquet® sauce

- ❑ mayonnaise, light
- ❑ Parmesan cheese
- ❑ peanut butter
- ❑ rice vinegar
- ❑ salsa
- ❑ soy sauce, low-sodium
- ❑ Worcestershire sauce

Breads, Cereals and Pasta
- ❑ croutons, fat-free seasoned
- ❑ egg noodles
- ❑ English muffin
- ❑ flour tortillas
- ❑ French bread
- ❑ Grape Nuts® cereal
- ❑ lasagna noodles
- ❑ oatmeal, instant
- ❑ puffed rice cereal
- ❑ soba noodles
- ❑ sourdough bread
- ❑ spaghetti

Canned/Frozen Foods
- ❑ beef broth
- ❑ black beans
- ❑ black olives, sliced
- ❑ chicken broth, fat-free, lower-sodium
- ❑ chopped broccoli, frozen
- ❑ chopped spinach, frozen
- ❑ corn
- ❑ cream of celery soup, condensed, reduced-fat, reduced-sodium
- ❑ cream of mushroom soup, 98% fat free
- ❑ frozen broccoli (or spinach)
- ❑ frozen mixed vegetables
- ❑ garlic cloves, minced
- ❑ green peas, frozen
- ❑ pimentoes, diced
- ❑ sliced mushrooms

- ❑ tomato paste
- ❑ tomatoes
- ❑ tomatoes, crushed
- ❑ tomatoes, diced with juice
- ❑ tuna, in water
- ❑ vegetable broth

Dairy Products
- ❑ butter
- ❑ cheddar cheese, 2%
- ❑ cottage cheese, 1% fat
- ❑ margarine, light
- ❑ margarine, stick
- ❑ milk, nonfat
- ❑ Monterey Jack cheese
- ❑ mozzarella cheese
- ❑ provolone or mozzarella cheese
- ❑ sour cream, low-fat
- ❑ whipped topping, fat-free frozen
- ❑ yogurt, fat free
- ❑ yogurt, low-fat vanilla

Juices
- ❑ lemon juice
- ❑ lime juice

Meat and Poultry
- ❑ chicken breast, rotisserie
- ❑ chicken breasts, skinless, boneless
- ❑ egg substitute
- ❑ eggs
- ❑ ground beef, lean
- ❑ grouper (or other white fish fillets)
- ❑ ham
- ❑ pork chops, bone-in center-cut loin
- ❑ shrimp, medium
- ❑ top round steak
- ❑ turkey breast

Second Week Meals and Recipes

DAY 1

Breakfast

Chocolate Peanut Butter Smoothie

½ cup low-fat milk
2 tbsp. chocolate syrup
2 tbsp. creamy peanut butter

1 frozen sliced ripe banana
1 (8-oz.) carton vanilla low-fat
  yogurt

Place all ingredients in a blender; process until smooth. Serves 2.

Nutritional Information: 332 calories; 10.8g fat; 12.7g protein; 49.8g carbohydrate; 3.1g dietary fiber; 8mg cholesterol; 194mg sodium.

Lunch

Easy Vegetable Soup

1 bag (32 oz.) frozen mixed vegetables
2 cans beef broth
1 can vegetable broth
1 can fat-free, lower-sodium chicken
  broth
1 (15-oz.) can diced tomatoes

4 medium red potatoes, cut into
  pieces
½ bag (½ lb.) carrots, sliced
¼ head cabbage, sliced
1 medium onion, chopped
basil and bay leaf, to taste

Mix all ingredients together in large pot. Simmer until vegetables are tender (about 20 minutes). Remove bay leaves before serving. Serves 10.

Nutritional Information: 120 calories; 1g fat; 8g protein; 20g carbohydrate; 3g dietary fiber; trace cholesterol; 876mg sodium.

Dinner

Vegetable Lasagna

2 tbsp. olive oil
½ cup onion, diced
1 tbsp. garlic, chopped
1½ tbsp. Italian seasoning
½ tsp. basil
1 tsp. salt
1 tsp. black pepper

1 (28-oz.) can crushed tomatoes
1 (14-oz.) can diced tomatoes
1 (6-oz.) can tomato paste
5 cups vegetables, chopped
12 lasagna noodles
1 (10-oz.) box chopped spinach,
  thawed

3 cups mozzarella cheese, grated
16 oz. (1% fat) cottage cheese

6 tbsp. Parmesan cheese, grated
nonstick cooking spray

In 6-quart stock pot, sauté onion and garlic in oil until tender. Add seasonings, canned tomatoes and paste. Cover and simmer 40 minutes, stirring occasionally. Chop 4 to 6 cups assorted vegetables (you can use broccoli, cauliflower, yellow and zucchini squash, bell peppers, mushrooms, carrots, red onions or whatever you like). Add chopped vegetables to sauce mixture for the last 10 minutes and cook until vegetables are crisp tender. Set sauce aside. Boil 12 lasagna noodles according to package directions. Drain and set aside. Cook 1 box chopped spinach according to package directions. Drain, press out excess water, and set aside.

Spray bottom of 13" x 9" pan with nonstick cooking spray. Place 4 noodles across bottom of pan. Top with ⅓ of the sauce/vegetable mixture. Spread ⅓ of the cottage cheese on top and spread evenly. Sprinkle with ⅓ of the Parmesan cheese and top with ⅓ of mozzarella cheese. Spread entire box of spinach evenly over cheese. Repeat for noodles, vegetable and cheeses 2 more times, ending with mozzarella cheese on top. Bake at 350° F for 30 to 40 minutes or until light brown on top and bubbling on sides. Let stand 10 to 15 minutes before serving. Serves 12.

Nutritional Information: 284 calories; 9g fat; 19g protein; 33g carbohydrate; 3g dietary fiber; 19mg cholesterol; 678mg sodium.

DAY 2

Breakfast

⅓ medium cantaloupe
1 cup fat-free yogurt

¼ cup Grape Nuts® cereal (sprinkled over yogurt)

Nutritional Information: 281 calories; 1g fat; 15g protein; 57g carbohydrate; 5g dietary fiber; 3mg cholesterol; 345mg sodium

Lunch

Broccoli and Mushroom Quiche with Ham

1 prepared piecrust, unbaked
1 (10-oz.) box frozen chopped
   broccoli (or chopped spinach)
1 cup mushroom, sliced
½ cup onion, chopped
½ cup celery, chopped

1 tbsp. butter
3 eggs, slightly beaten
2 cups mozzarella cheese, grated
1 (10-oz.) can 98% fat-free cream of
   mushroom soup
4 oz. cooked ham, chopped

Cook broccoli as directed on package and drain. Sauté mushrooms, onion and celery in butter until tender. Combine all ingredients and pour into pie shell. Bake at 350° F for about 1 hour or until light brown on top. Let sit 15 minutes before cutting or serving. Serves 6.

Nutritional Information: 383 calories; 22g fat; 21g protein; 22g carbohydrate; 3g dietary fiber; 143mg cholesterol; 851mg sodium.

Dinner

Chicken Supreme

3 egg whites
6 (4-oz.) boneless, skinless chicken breasts, pounded flat
¾ cup breadcrumbs
¾ cup Parmesan cheese, grated

1 tsp. salt and ¼ tsp. black pepper
2 tbsp. parsley
1 garlic clove, minced
¼ oz. slivered almonds
nonstick cooking spray

Preheat oven to 350° F. Slightly beat egg whites in small bowl; set aside. In shallow dish, combine breadcrumbs, cheese, salt, pepper, parsley, garlic and almonds (reserve a few almonds for garnish). Dip chicken breasts in egg whites, roll in breadcrumb mixture, and arrange in 9″ x 13″ baking dish sprayed with nonstick cooking spray. Garnish with a few almond slivers. Bake 20-30 minutes or until golden brown. Top with *Mushroom Gravy* (see recipe below). Serves 6.

Nutritional Information: 294 calories; 17g fat; 22g protein; 12g carbohydrate; 1g dietary fiber; 83mg cholesterol; 1,024mg sodium.

Mushroom Gravy

¼ cup light margarine
2 cups sliced mushrooms
1 cup fat-free, lower-sodium chicken broth (or vegetable broth)

2 tsp. cornstarch
1 tsp. salt
black pepper, to taste
1 tsp. Kitchen Bouquet® sauce

In medium skillet, sauté mushrooms in melted margarine over medium heat. Gradually add broth to mushrooms and continue to stir. Dissolve cornstarch in small amount of water. Add to the mushroom mixture, stirring constantly until thickened. Add seasonings to taste and a small amount of Kitchen Bouquet to color. Spoon over the cooked chicken breasts and serve. Serves 6.

Nutritional Information: 55 calories; 5g fat; 2g protein; 12g carbohydrate; 1g dietary fiber; trace cholesterol; 694mg sodium.

DAY 3

Breakfast

1 (2-oz.) English muffin
1 tsp. light margarine

½ medium grapefruit
1 cup nonfat milk

Nutritional Information: 273 calories; 3g fat; 13g protein; 48g carbohydrate; 3g dietary fiber; 4mg cholesterol; 435mg sodium.

Lunch

Shrimp Caesar Salad

Dressing:

2 tbsp. light mayonnaise
2 tbsp. water
2 tbsp. lemon juice
1 tsp. Parmesan cheese, grated

¼ tsp. black pepper
¼ tsp. chili sauce
⅛ tsp. Worcestershire sauce
2 garlic cloves, minced

Salad:

¾ cup fat-free seasoned croutons
2 tbsp. Parmesan cheese, grated
1½ lbs. medium shrimp, cooked and
 peeled

1 (10-oz.) package romaine lettuce,
 chopped
3 tbsp. pine nuts, toasted
fresh chives, chopped (optional)

To prepare dressing, combine mayonnaise, water, lemon juice, Parmesan cheese, black pepper, chili sauce, Worcestershire sauce and garlic cloves. Stir with a whisk. To prepare salad, combine croutons, cheese, shrimp and lettuce in a large bowl. Add dressing; toss well to coat. Top with pine nuts. Garnish with chives, if desired. Serve immediately. Serves 4.

Nutritional Information: 295 calories; 9.4g fat; 38.6g protein; 12.2g carbohydrate; 1.8g dietary fiber; 261mg cholesterol; 462mg sodium.

Dinner

Baked Spaghetti Casserole

1 cup onion, chopped
1 cup bell pepper, chopped
2 tsp. garlic, chopped
1 cup mushrooms, sliced
1 lb. lean ground beef
1 (28-oz.) can diced tomatoes
2¼ oz. can sliced black olives

2 tsp. oregano
12 oz. spaghetti, cooked and drained
2 cups (2%) cheddar cheese, grated
1 (10¾-oz.) can 98% fat-free cream
 of mushroom soup, mixed with
 ¼ cup water
¼ cup Parmesan cheese

In a Dutch oven, combine onion, peppers, mushrooms, meat and garlic; cook until meat is browned and onion is tender. Skim off excess fat. Add tomatoes, olives and oregano. Simmer uncovered for 10 minutes. Place half of the spaghetti into a greased 13″ x 9″ x 2″ baking dish. Top with half of the meat mixture and 1 cup cheese. Repeat layers of spaghetti, meat and cheese. Top with soup mixture and sprinkle top with Parmesan cheese. Bake at 350° F for 30 to 45 minutes or until bubbly. Freezes well. Serves 12.

Nutritional Information: 464 calories; 22g fat; 21g protein; 48g carbohydrate; 5g dietary fiber; 64mg cholesterol; 595mg sodium.

Serve with a tossed salad and light dressing.

DAY 4

Breakfast

1 package instant unflavored oatmeal topped with 4 walnut halves, chopped	½ banana 1 cup nonfat milk

Nutritional Information: 439 calories; 6g fat; 22g protein; 78g carbohydrate; 10g dietary fiber; 4mg cholesterol; 945mg sodium.

Lunch

Turkey and Cheese Panini

2 tbsp. light mayonnaise	2 oz. provolone or mozzarella cheese, thinly sliced
4 tsp. basil pesto	8 (⅛″ thick) slices tomato
8 (1-oz.) pieces sourdough bread, thinly sliced	nonstick cooking spray
8 oz. cooked turkey breast, sliced	

Combine mayonnaise and pesto, stirring well. Spread 1 tablespoon of the mayonnaise mixture on each of 4 bread slices; top each slice with 2 ounces turkey, ½ ounce cheese, and 2 tomato slices. Top with remaining bread slices. Preheat grill pan or large nonstick skillet coated with nonstick cooking spray over medium heat. Add sandwiches to pan; top with another heavy skillet. Cook 3 minutes on each side or until golden brown. (Using a grill skillet will give the sandwich appetizing grill marks, but the recipe works just as well in a regular nonstick skillet.) Serves 4.

Nutritional Information: 257 calories; 8.2g fat; 18.4g protein; 30.4g carbohydrate; 4.1g dietary fiber; 30mg cholesterol; 1,208mg sodium.

Dinner

Easy Baked Fish

1½ lbs. grouper/other white fish fillets
1 tbsp. lime juice
1 tbsp. light mayonnaise
⅛ tsp. onion powder
⅛ tsp. black pepper

½ cup breadcrumbs
1½ tbsp. butter or light margarine,
  melted
2 tbsp. fresh parsley, chopped
nonstick cooking spray

Preheat oven to 425° F. Place fish in an 11" x 7" baking dish coated with nonstick cooking spray. Combine lime juice, mayonnaise, onion powder and pepper in a small bowl and spread over fish. Sprinkle with breadcrumbs; drizzle with butter. Bake at 425° F for 20 minutes or until fish flakes easily when tested with a fork. Sprinkle with parsley. (*Note*: Haddock or cod would make good substitutes for the grouper. Adjust the baking time depending on the thickness of the fish.) Serves 4.

Nutritional Information: 223 calories; 7.5g fat; 33.6g protein; 5.3g carbohydrate; 0.2g dietary fiber; 84mg cholesterol; 223mg sodium.

Serve with roasted potatoes and fresh steamed vegetables.

DAY 5

Breakfast

1 cup puffed rice cereal
1 cup nonfat milk

½ banana, sliced

Nutritional Information: 194 calories; 1g fat; 10g protein; 38g carbohydrate; 2g dietary fiber; 4mg cholesterol; 127mg sodium.

Lunch

Chicken and Bean Burrito

¼ cup water
2 tbsp. lime juice
½ tsp. chili powder
¼ tsp. ground cumin
¼ tsp. black pepper
⅛ tsp. ground red pepper
2 cups rotisserie chicken breast,
  shredded

¼ cup green onions, thinly sliced
¾ cup canned black beans, rinsed
  and drained
½ cup salsa
4 (8") flour tortillas
½ cup Monterey Jack cheese,
  shredded
nonstick cooking spray

Bring water, lime juice and seasonings to a boil in a small saucepan. Stir in shredded chicken and green onions. In a separate bowl, combine beans and salsa. Spoon ¼ cup bean mixture and ½ cup chicken mixture down center of each tortilla; sprinkle with 2 tablespoons cheese. Roll up. Heat a large skillet over medium-high heat. Coat pan with nonstick cooking spray. Add 2 burritos. Place a cast-iron or other heavy skillet on top of burritos and cook for 3 minutes on each side. Remove from pan and repeat procedure with the remaining 2 burritos. Serves 4.

Nutritional Information: 353 calories; 9.8g fat; 30.9g protein; 33.1g carbohydrate; 2.4g dietary fiber; 72mg cholesterol; 595mg sodium.

Dinner
Barbequed Rubbed Pork Chops

1 tbsp. light brown sugar	¼ tsp. dry mustard
1 tsp. salt	⅛ tsp. ground allspice
1 tsp. paprika	⅛ tsp. ground red pepper
1 tsp. chili powder	4 (6-oz.) bone-in center-cut loin pork
¾ tsp. garlic powder	chops, trimmed (about ½" thick)
¾ tsp. ground cumin	nonstick cooking spray

Combine brown sugar, salt, paprika, chili powder, garlic powder, ground cumin, dry mustard, allspice and red pepper. Rub over both sides of pork. Heat a grill pan over medium-high heat. Coat pan with nonstick cooking spray. Add pork; cook for 2 minutes on each side. Reduce heat to medium and cook for 8 minutes or until done, turning occasionally. Remove from pan; let stand 5 minutes. Serves 4.

Nutritional Information: 277 calories; 10.5g fat; 38.86g protein; 4.3g carbohydrate; 0.5g dietary fiber; 105mg cholesterol; 669mg sodium.

DAY 6

Breakfast
½ toasted English muffin topped with 1 tbsp. peanut butter and ½ banana
1 cup nonfat milk

Nutritional Information: 302 calories; 9g fat; 15g protein; 42g carbohydrate; 3g dietary fiber; 4mg cholesterol; 334mg sodium.

Lunch

Asian Chicken Salad

2 cups water	½ tsp. salt
2 (6-oz.) skinless, boneless chicken breast halves	2 cups cooked soba noodles (about 4 oz. uncooked)
4 black peppercorns	1 cup grated carrot
1 bay leaf, dried	½ cup green onions, thinly sliced
1 tbsp. rice vinegar	¼ cup red onion, minced
2 tbsp. roasted peanut oil	¼ cup fresh basil, chopped
2 tsp. low-sodium soy sauce	4 tsp. unsalted, dry-roasted peanuts, chopped
1 tsp. honey	lime wedges (optional)
1 tsp. chili sauce	

Combine water, chicken, peppercorns and bay leaf in a medium saucepan; bring to a boil. Cover, remove from heat, and let stand 15 minutes or until chicken is done. Remove chicken from pan and discard peppercorns, bay leaf and cooking liquid. Shred chicken; place in a large bowl. (For convenience, you may also use 12 ounces pre-cooked rotisserie chicken.) Combine vinegar, peanut oil, soy sauce, honey, chili sauce and salt, stirring with a whisk. Pour over chicken; let stand 5 minutes. Add soba noodles, carrots, green and red onions and basil to chicken mixture, and toss well. Sprinkle with peanuts. Garnish with lime wedges, if desired. Serves 4.

Nutritional Information: 256 calories; 9.5g fat; 23.9g protein; 19.5g carbohydrate; 2.5g dietary fiber; 49mg cholesterol; 538mg sodium.

Dinner

Crock Pot Beef Stroganoff

1 lb. top round steak (1″ thick), trimmed	8-oz. package sliced mushrooms (about 2 cups)
1 cup onion, chopped	3 garlic cloves, minced
2 tbsp. fresh parsley, chopped	⅓ cup all-purpose flour
2 tbsp. Dijon mustard	1 cup beef broth
¾ tsp. salt	1 (8-oz.) container low-fat sour cream
½ tsp. dried dill	2 cups hot cooked medium egg noodles (about 4 oz. uncooked)
½ tsp. black pepper	

Cut steak diagonally across grain into ¼-inch thick slices. Place steak, onion, parsley, mustard, salt, dill, pepper, mushrooms and garlic in a 3-quart electric slow cooker; stir well. Spoon flour into a dry measuring cup; level with a knife. Place flour in a small bowl; gradually add broth, stirring with a whisk until blended. Add broth mixture to slow cooker; stir well. Cover with lid; cook on high-heat setting 1 hour. Reduce to low-heat setting and cook 7 to 8 hours or until steak is tender. Turn slow cooker off; remove lid. Let stand 10 minutes. Stir in sour cream. Serve stroganoff over noodles. Serves 4.

Nutritional Information: 404 calories; 10.1g fat; 35.8g protein; 43.2g carbohydrate; 2.9g dietary fiber; 113mg cholesterol; 946mg sodium.

DAY 7

Breakfast
French Toast Casserole

²⁄₃ cup packed dark brown sugar
2 tbsp. butter
2 tbsp. dark corn syrup
1½ cups low-fat milk
½ cup egg substitute
1 tsp. vanilla extract
¼ tsp. salt
⅛ tsp. orange rind, grated
2 large eggs

6 (1½" thick) slices French bread
6 tbsp. frozen fat-free whipped topping, thawed
1 to 2 tsp. Grand Marnier (orange-flavored liqueur), optional
2 tbsp. finely chopped pecans, toasted
nonstick cooking spray

Combine brown sugar, butter and corn syrup in a small, heavy saucepan over medium heat. Cook 5 minutes or until bubbly and sugar dissolves, stirring constantly. Pour sugar mixture into bottom of a 13" x 9" baking dish coated with cooking spray. Spread mixture evenly over bottom of pan. Set aside; cool completely. Combine milk, egg substitute, vanilla, salt orange rind and eggs in a large shallow bowl; stir with a whisk. Dip 1 bread slice in milk mixture; arrange bread slice over sugar mixture in dish. Repeat procedure with remaining 5 bread slices. Pour any remaining egg mixture over bread slices. Cover and refrigerate overnight. Preheat oven to 350° F. Bake for 30 minutes or until lightly browned. While casserole bakes, combine whipped topping and Grand Marnier. Place 1 bread slice, caramel side up, on each of 6 plates; top each serving with 1 tablespoon topping and 1 teaspoon pecans. Serves 6. (*Note*: French bread with a soft crust works best because it is easier to cut. Omit the liqueur in the whipped topping, if you prefer. Garnish with fresh strawberries or an orange slice.)

Nutritional Information: 352 calories; 8.8g fat; 11.1g protein; 58.1g carbohydrate; 1.2g dietary fiber; 83mg cholesterol; 466mg sodium.

Lunch

Spicy Chicken Corn Soup

1 tbsp. olive oil
1¾ cups onion, chopped
3 garlic cloves, minced
1 jalapeño pepper, seeded and
  minced
2 cups shredded skinless, boneless
  rotisserie chicken breast

¼ tsp. black pepper
2 (14-oz.) cans fat-free, lower-sodium
  chicken broth
1 (15½-oz.) can corn, drained
½ cup radishes, thinly sliced
2 tbsp. fresh cilantro leaves
4 lime wedges

Heat olive oil in a large saucepan over medium-high heat. Add onion to pan; sauté 2 minutes. Stir in garlic and jalapeño; sauté 1 minute. Add chicken, black pepper and broth; bring to a boil. Reduce heat and simmer 5 minutes. Stir in corn; bring to a boil. Cook 5 minutes. Ladle about 1½ cups soup into each of 4 bowls; top each serving with 2 tablespoons radishes and 1½ teaspoons cilantro. Serve with lime wedges. Serves 4.

Nutritional Information: 235 calories; 6.6g fat; 24.8g protein; 18g carbohydrate; 3.3g dietary fiber; 60mg cholesterol; 641mg sodium.

Dinner

Easy Tuna Casserole

1 cup fresh mushrooms, sliced
1 cup onion, chopped
⅓ cup celery, sliced
1 small garlic clove, minced
¾ cup low-fat milk
¼ cup Parmesan cheese, grated
¼ cup light mayonnaise
½ tsp. dried dill
¼ tsp. salt
¼ tsp. black pepper
3½ cups cooked medium egg noodles
  (about 2¼ cups uncooked)

1 (10¾ -oz.) can reduced-fat, reduced-
  sodium condensed cream of celery
  soup, undiluted
1 cup frozen green peas
1 (9¼-oz.) can tuna in water,
  drained
1 (2-oz.) jar diced pimento, drained
¼ cup breadcrumbs
¼ cup Parmesan cheese, grated
1 tbsp. margarine, melted
nonstick cooking spray

Coat a large nonstick skillet with nonstick cooking spray, and place over medium heat until hot. Add mushrooms, onion, celery and garlic; sauté for 6 minutes or until tender. Combine milk, Parmesan cheese, mayonnaise, dill, salt, pepper and cream of celery soup in a bowl; stir well. Add mushroom mixture, noodles, peas, tuna and pimento; stir gently. Spoon noodle mixture into a shallow 2-quart casserole coated with nonstick cooking spray. Cover and bake at 350° F for 40 minutes. Combine the breadcrumbs, Parmesan cheese and margarine in a small bowl; stir well and sprinkle over casserole. Bake, uncovered, at 350° F for 10 minutes. (*Note:* You can assemble the casserole up to 4 hours ahead of time, omitting breadcrumb mixture; cover and chill.) Let stand at room temperature 30 minutes before baking. Top with breadcrumb mixture during last 10 minutes of baking. Serves 6.

DESSERTS
(Note: You will need to add these items to the grocery list)

Banana-split Dessert

24 low-fat graham crackers
2 (1.3 oz.) boxes vanilla, sugar-free instant pudding
4½ cups nonfat milk, divided
1 (16-oz.) can crushed pineapple, drained well

3 cups Cool Whip Lite®, thawed
2 bananas
2 cups sliced strawberries
1 (1.3-oz.) box sugar-free, chocolate-flavored instant pudding
2 tbsp. pecans, chopped

Line bottom of 13″ x 9″ baking dish with 8 graham crackers; set aside. In large bowl, combine vanilla pudding mix and 3 cups milk; mix well and let sit 2 minutes. Stir in crushed pineapple, and then gently fold in whipped topping. Pour half the mixture into baking dish; reserve remainder. Arrange banana slices over pudding mixture; add layer of 8 graham crackers. Pour in remaining pudding mixture; add layer of sliced strawberries and top with remaining graham crackers. Set aside. In separate bowl, combine chocolate pudding mix with 1½ cups milk; mix well and let sit 2 minutes. Spread as topping over graham crackers. Refrigerate at least 6 hours to soften graham crackers; garnish with chopped pecans prior to serving. Serves 18.

Nutritional Information: 145 calories; 3g fat; 4g protein; 27g carbohydrate; 1g dietary fiber; 1mg cholesterol; 222mg sodium.

Orange Amaretto Dessert

¼ cup Cool Whip Lite®
1 amaretto cookie, crushed

¾ cup orange sherbet, softened
2 amaretto cookies

Fold whipped topping and crushed cookie into sherbet. Pipe or spoon into 2 dessert dishes. Serve each immediately with one cookie. Serves 2.

Nutritional Information: 168 calories; 5.3g fat; 1.6g protein; 30.5g carbohydrates; 0.3g dietary fiber; 4mg cholesterol; 92mg sodium.

Creamy Pumpkin Pie

1 prepared reduced-fat graham
   cracker pie crust
1 (1.3-oz.) box sugar-free, vanilla-
   flavored instant pudding
1 cup nonfat milk

1 (16-oz.) can pumpkin
½ tsp. nutmeg
½ tsp. ginger
½ tsp. cinnamon
1 cup Cool Whip Lite®

Combine pudding mix and milk in medium bowl; stir well (will be very thick). Add pumpkin, nutmeg, ginger and cinnamon; mix well. Gently fold in whipped topping; pour into pie shell. Chill for one hour or until set. Top with additional dollop of topping. Serves 8.

Nutritional Information: 156 calories; 6g fat; 1g protein; 14g carbohydrate; 1g dietary fiber; 1mg cholesterol; 115mg sodium.

Lemon Bars

¾ cup flour
3 tbsp. sugar
¼ cup margarine
1 egg
1 egg white
⅔ cup granulated sugar
2 tbsp. flour

¼ tsp. lemon peel, finely
   shredded
2 tbsp. lemon juice
1 tbsp. water
¼ tsp. baking powder
1 tbsp. powdered sugar
nonstick cooking spray

Spray an 8″ x 8″ x 2″ baking pan with nonstick cooking spray. In a small mixing bowl, combine ¾ cup flour with 3 tablespoons sugar. Cut in margarine till crumbly. Pat mixture into bottom of prepared pan. Bake at 350° F for 15 minutes. Meanwhile, in the same bowl combine egg and egg white. Beat with an electric mixer on medium speed until frothy. Add ⅔ cup sugar, 2 tablespoons flour, lemon peel, juice, water and baking powder. Beat on medium speed until slightly thickened. Pour mixture over baked layer in pan. Bake for 20 to 25 minutes more or until edges are light brown and center is set. Cool in pan on a wire rack. Sift powdered sugar over top. Cut into bars. Store left over bars in refrigerator. Serves 9.

Nutritional Information: 177 calories; 6g fat; 2g protein; 30g carbohydrate; trace dietary fiber; 24mg cholesterol; 87mg sodium.

Member Survey

Please answer the following questions to help your leader plan your First Place 4 Health meetings so that your needs might be met in this session. Give this form to your leader at the first group meeting.

Name _____ Birth date _____

Please list those who live in your household.

Name	Relationship	Age
_____	_____	_____
_____	_____	_____
_____	_____	_____
_____	_____	_____

What church do you attend? _____

Are you interested in receiving more information about our church?

        Yes   No

Occupation _____

What talent or area of expertise would you be willing to share with our class?

_____

Why did you join First Place 4 Health?

_____

With notice, would you be willing to lead a Bible study discussion one week?

        Yes   No

Are you comfortable praying out loud? _____

If the assistant leader were absent, would you be willing to assist in weighing in members and possibly evaluating the Live It Trackers?

        Yes   No

Any other comments:

_____

_____

Personal Weight and Measurement Record

Week	Weight	+ or -	Goal this Session	Pounds to goal
1				
2				
3				
4				
5				
6				
7				
8				
9				
10				
11				
12				

Beginning Measurements

Waist _____ Hips _____ Thighs _____ Chest _____

Ending Measurements

Waist _____ Hips _____ Thighs _____ Chest _____

First Place 4 Health
Prayer Partner

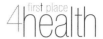

MOTIVATED TO
WELLNESS
Week
1

SCRIPTURE VERSE TO MEMORIZE FOR WEEK TWO:

Blessed is the man who makes the LORD his trust, who does not look to the proud, to those who turn aside to false gods.

PSALM 40:4

Date: _____

Name: _____

Home Phone: (_____) _____

Work Phone: (_____) _____

Email: _____

Personal Prayer Concerns:

_____

_____

_____

_____

_____

_____

_____

This form is for prayer requests that are personal to you and your journey in First Place 4 Health. Please complete this form and have it ready to turn in when you arrive at your group meeting.

First Place 4 Health
Prayer Partner

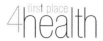

MOTIVATED TO
WELLNESS
Week
2

Date: _____

Name: _____

Home Phone: (____) _____

Work Phone: (____) _____

Email: _____

Personal Prayer Concerns:

_____

_____

_____

_____

_____

_____

_____

This form is for prayer requests that are personal to you and your journey in First Place 4 Health. Please complete this form and have it ready to turn in when you arrive at your group meeting.

First Place 4 Health
Prayer Partner

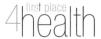

SCRIPTURE VERSE TO MEMORIZE FOR WEEK FOUR:

See, I am doing a new thing! Now it springs up; do you not perceive it?
I am making a way in the desert and streams in the wasteland.

ISAIAH 43:19

Date: _____

Name: _____

Home Phone: (_____) _____

Work Phone: (_____) _____

Email: _____

Personal Prayer Concerns:

_____

_____

_____

_____

_____

_____

_____

This form is for prayer requests that are personal to you and your journey in First Place 4 Health. Please complete this form and have it ready to turn in when you arrive at your group meeting.

First Place 4 Health
Prayer Partner

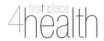

MOTIVATED TO
WELLNESS
Week
4

SCRIPTURE VERSE TO MEMORIZE FOR WEEK FIVE:

Let us not become weary in doing good, for at the proper time we will reap a harvest if we do not give up.

GALATIANS 6:9

Date: _____

Name: _____

Home Phone: (_____) _____

Work Phone: (_____) _____

Email: _____

Personal Prayer Concerns:

_____

_____

_____

_____

_____

_____

_____

This form is for prayer requests that are personal to you and your journey in First Place 4 Health. Please complete this form and have it ready to turn in when you arrive at your group meeting.

First Place 4 Health
Prayer Partner

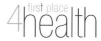

MOTIVATED TO
WELLNESS
Week
5

SCRIPTURE VERSE TO MEMORIZE FOR WEEK SIX:

*My eyes stay open through the watches of the night,
that I may meditate on your promises.*

PSALM 119:148

Date: _____

Name: _____

Home Phone: (_____) _____

Work Phone: (_____) _____

Email: _____

Personal Prayer Concerns:

_____

_____

_____

_____

_____

_____

_____

This form is for prayer requests that are personal to you and your journey in First Place 4 Health. Please complete this form and have it ready to turn in when you arrive at your group meeting.

First Place 4 Health
Prayer Partner

MOTIVATED TO
WELLNESS
Week
6

SCRIPTURE VERSE TO MEMORIZE FOR WEEK SEVEN:

Look to the LORD and his strength; seek his face always.

PSALM 105:4

Date: _____

Name: _____

Home Phone: (_____) _____

Work Phone: (_____) _____

Email: _____

Personal Prayer Concerns:

_____

_____

_____

_____

_____

_____

_____

This form is for prayer requests that are personal to you and your journey in First Place 4 Health. Please complete this form and have it ready to turn in when you arrive at your group meeting.

First Place 4 Health
Prayer Partner

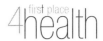

MOTIVATED TO
WELLNESS
Week
7

Date: _____

Name: _____

Home Phone: (_____) _____

Work Phone: (_____) _____

Email: _____

Personal Prayer Concerns:

_____

_____

_____

_____

_____

_____

_____

This form is for prayer requests that are personal to you and your journey in First Place 4 Health. Please complete this form and have it ready to turn in when you arrive at your group meeting.

First Place 4 Health
Prayer Partner

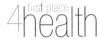

Scripture Verse to Memorize for Week Nine:

Be strong and take heart, all you who hope in the Lord.

Psalm 31:24

Date: _____

Name: _____

Home Phone: (_____) _____

Work Phone: (_____) _____

Email: _____

Personal Prayer Concerns:

_____

_____

_____

_____

_____

_____

_____

_____

This form is for prayer requests that are personal to you and your journey in First Place 4 Health. Please complete this form and have it ready to turn in when you arrive at your group meeting.

First Place 4 Health
Prayer Partner

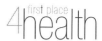

Scripture Verse to Memorize for Week Ten:

*Enlarge the place of your tent, stretch your tent curtains wide,
do not hold back; lengthen your cords, strengthen your stakes.*

Isaiah 54:2

Date: _____

Name: _____

Home Phone: (_____) _____

Work Phone: (_____) _____

Email: _____

Personal Prayer Concerns:

_____

_____

_____

_____

_____

_____

_____

This form is for prayer requests that are personal to you and your journey in First Place 4 Health. Please complete this form and have it ready to turn in when you arrive at your group meeting.

First Place 4 Health
Prayer Partner

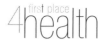

SCRIPTURE VERSE TO MEMORIZE FOR WEEK ELEVEN:

Now devote your heart and soul to seeking the LORD your God.

1 CHRONICLES 22:19

Date: _____

Name: _____

Home Phone: (_____) _____

Work Phone: (_____) _____

Email: _____

Personal Prayer Concerns:

_____

_____

_____

_____

_____

_____

_____

_____

This form is for prayer requests that are personal to you and your journey in First Place 4 Health. Please complete this form and have it ready to turn in when you arrive at your group meeting.

First Place 4 Health
Prayer Partner

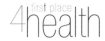

MOTIVATED TO
WELLNESS
Week
11

Date: _____

Name: _____

Home Phone: (_____) _____

Work Phone: (_____) _____

Email: _____

Personal Prayer Concerns:

_____

_____

_____

_____

_____

_____

_____

This form is for prayer requests that are personal to you and your journey in First Place 4 Health. Please complete this form and have it ready to turn in when you arrive at your group meeting.

Live It Tracker

Name: _____ Date: _____ Week #: _____

Loss/gain _____ lbs. Calorie Range: _____ My food goal for the week: _____

_____

Activity Level: None, < 30 min/day, 30-60 min/day, 60+ min/day My activity goal for the week: _____

My spiritual goal for the week: _____

Group	Daily Calories							
	1300-1400	1500-1600	1700-1800	1900-2000	2100-2200	2300-2400	2500-2600	2700-2800
Fruits	1.5-2 c.	1.5-2 c.	1.5-2 c.	2-2.5 c.	2-2.5 c.	2.5-3.5 c.	3.5-4.5 c.	3.5-4.5 c.
Vegetables	1.5-2 c.	2-2.5 c.	2.5-3 c.	2.5-3 c.	3-3.5 c.	3.5-4.5 c.	4.5-5 c.	4.5-5 c.
Grains	5 oz-eq.	5-6 oz-eq.	6-7 oz-eq.	6-7 oz-eq.	7-8 oz-eq.	8-9 oz-eq.	9-10 oz-eq.	10-11 oz-eq.
Meat & Beans	4 oz-eq.	5 oz-eq.	5-5.5 oz-eq.	5.5-6.5 oz-eq.	6.5-7 oz-eq.	7-7.5 oz-eq.	7-7.5 oz-eq.	7.5-8 oz-eq.
Milk	2-3 c.	3 c.	3 c.	3 c.	3 c.	3 c.	3 c.	3 c.
Healthy Oils	4 tsp.	5 tsp.	5 tsp.	6 tsp.	6 tsp.	7 tsp.	8 tsp.	8 tsp.

Day/Date:

Breakfast: _____
Lunch: _____
Dinner: _____
Snacks: _____

GROUP	FRUITS	VEGETABLES	GRAINS	MEAT & BEANS	MILK	OILS
Goal Amount						
Estimate Your Total						
Total Calories						

Physical Activity: _____ Spiritual Activity: _____
Steps/Miles/Minutes: _____ My Emotions Today: ❏ Happy ❏ Sad ❏ Stressed

Day/Date:

Breakfast: _____
Lunch: _____
Dinner: _____
Snacks: _____

GROUP	FRUITS	VEGETABLES	GRAINS	MEAT & BEANS	MILK	OILS
Goal Amount						
Estimate Your Total						
Total Calories						

Physical Activity: _____ Spiritual Activity: _____
Steps/Miles/Minutes: _____ My Emotions Today: ❏ Happy ❏ Sad ❏ Stressed

Day/Date:

Breakfast: _____
Lunch: _____
Dinner: _____
Snacks: _____

GROUP	FRUITS	VEGETABLES	GRAINS	MEAT & BEANS	MILK	OILS
Goal Amount						
Estimate Your Total						
Total Calories						

Physical Activity: _____ Spiritual Activity: _____
Steps/Miles/Minutes: _____ My Emotions Today: ❏ Happy ❏ Sad ❏ Stressed

Day/Date:

Breakfast: _____

Lunch: _____

Dinner: _____

Snacks: _____

GROUP	FRUITS	VEGETABLES	GRAINS	MEAT & BEANS	MILK	OILS
Goal Amount						
Estimate Your Total						
Total Calories						

Physical Activity: _____ Spiritual Activity: _____

Steps/Miles/Minutes: _____ My Emotions Today: ❑ Happy   ❑ Sad   ❑ Stressed

---

Day/Date:

Breakfast: _____

Lunch: _____

Dinner: _____

Snacks: _____

GROUP	FRUITS	VEGETABLES	GRAINS	MEAT & BEANS	MILK	OILS
Goal Amount						
Estimate Your Total						
Total Calories						

Physical Activity: _____ Spiritual Activity: _____

Steps/Miles/Minutes: _____ My Emotions Today: ❑ Happy   ❑ Sad   ❑ Stressed

---

Day/Date:

Breakfast: _____

Lunch: _____

Dinner: _____

Snacks: _____

GROUP	FRUITS	VEGETABLES	GRAINS	MEAT & BEANS	MILK	OILS
Goal Amount						
Estimate Your Total						
Total Calories						

Physical Activity: _____ Spiritual Activity: _____

Steps/Miles/Minutes: _____ My Emotions Today: ❑ Happy   ❑ Sad   ❑ Stressed

---

Day/Date:

Breakfast: _____

Lunch: _____

Dinner: _____

Snacks: _____

GROUP	FRUITS	VEGETABLES	GRAINS	MEAT & BEANS	MILK	OILS
Goal Amount						
Estimate Your Total						
Total Calories						

Physical Activity: _____ Spiritual Activity: _____

Steps/Miles/Minutes: _____ My Emotions Today: ❑ Happy   ❑ Sad   ❑ Stressed

Live It Tracker

Name: _____   Date: _____   Week #: _____

Loss/gain _____ lbs.   Calorie Range: _____   My food goal for the week: _____

Activity Level: None, < 30 min/day, 30-60 min/day, 60+ min/day My activity goal for the week: _____

My spiritual goal for the week: _____

Group	Daily Calories							
	1300-1400	1500-1600	1700-1800	1900-2000	2100-2200	2300-2400	2500-2600	2700-2800
Fruits	1.5-2 c.	1.5-2 c.	1.5-2 c.	2-2.5 c.	2-2.5 c.	2.5-3.5 c.	3.5-4.5 c.	3.5-4.5 c.
Vegetables	1.5-2 c.	2-2.5 c.	2.5-3 c.	2.5-3 c.	3-3.5 c.	3.5-4.5 c.	4.5-5 c.	4.5-5 c.
Grains	5 oz-eq.	5-6 oz-eq.	6-7 oz-eq.	6-7 oz-eq.	7-8 oz-eq.	8-9 oz-eq.	9-10 oz-eq.	10-11 oz-eq.
Meat & Beans	4 oz-eq.	5 oz-eq.	5-5.5 oz-eq.	5.5-6.5 oz-eq.	6.5-7 oz-eq.	7-7.5 oz-eq.	7-7.5 oz-eq.	7.5-8 oz-eq.
Milk	2-3 c.	3 c.	3 c.	3 c.	3 c.	3 c.	3 c.	3 c.
Healthy Oils	4 tsp.	5 tsp.	5 tsp.	6 tsp.	6 tsp.	7 tsp.	8 tsp.	8 tsp.

Day/Date:

Breakfast: _____
Lunch: _____
Dinner: _____
Snacks: _____

GROUP	FRUITS	VEGETABLES	GRAINS	MEAT & BEANS	MILK	OILS
Goal Amount						
Estimate Your Total						
Total Calories						

Physical Activity: _____   Spiritual Activity: _____
Steps/Miles/Minutes: _____   My Emotions Today: ❑ Happy ❑ Sad ❑ Stressed

Day/Date:

Breakfast: _____
Lunch: _____
Dinner: _____
Snacks: _____

GROUP	FRUITS	VEGETABLES	GRAINS	MEAT & BEANS	MILK	OILS
Goal Amount						
Estimate Your Total						
Total Calories						

Physical Activity: _____   Spiritual Activity: _____
Steps/Miles/Minutes: _____   My Emotions Today: ❑ Happy ❑ Sad ❑ Stressed

Day/Date:

Breakfast: _____
Lunch: _____
Dinner: _____
Snacks: _____

GROUP	FRUITS	VEGETABLES	GRAINS	MEAT & BEANS	MILK	OILS
Goal Amount						
Estimate Your Total						
Total Calories						

Physical Activity: _____   Spiritual Activity: _____
Steps/Miles/Minutes: _____   My Emotions Today: ❑ Happy ❑ Sad ❑ Stressed

Day/Date:

Breakfast: _____
Lunch: _____
Dinner: _____
Snacks: _____

GROUP	FRUITS	VEGETABLES	GRAINS	MEAT & BEANS	MILK	OILS
Goal Amount						
Estimate Your Total						
Total Calories						

Physical Activity: _____   Spiritual Activity: _____
Steps/Miles/Minutes: _____   My Emotions Today: ❑ Happy ❑ Sad ❑ Stressed

Day/Date:

Breakfast: _____
Lunch: _____
Dinner: _____
Snacks: _____

GROUP	FRUITS	VEGETABLES	GRAINS	MEAT & BEANS	MILK	OILS
Goal Amount						
Estimate Your Total						
Total Calories						

Physical Activity: _____   Spiritual Activity: _____
Steps/Miles/Minutes: _____   My Emotions Today: ❑ Happy ❑ Sad ❑ Stressed

Day/Date:

Breakfast: _____
Lunch: _____
Dinner: _____
Snacks: _____

GROUP	FRUITS	VEGETABLES	GRAINS	MEAT & BEANS	MILK	OILS
Goal Amount						
Estimate Your Total						
Total Calories						

Physical Activity: _____   Spiritual Activity: _____
Steps/Miles/Minutes: _____   My Emotions Today: ❑ Happy ❑ Sad ❑ Stressed

Day/Date:

Breakfast: _____
Lunch: _____
Dinner: _____
Snacks: _____

GROUP	FRUITS	VEGETABLES	GRAINS	MEAT & BEANS	MILK	OILS
Goal Amount						
Estimate Your Total						
Total Calories						

Physical Activity: _____   Spiritual Activity: _____
Steps/Miles/Minutes: _____   My Emotions Today: ❑ Happy ❑ Sad ❑ Stressed

Live It Tracker

Name: _____ Date: _____ Week #: _____

Loss/gain _____ lbs.　Calorie Range: _____　My food goal for the week: _____

Activity Level:　None,　< 30 min/day,　30-60 min/day,　60+ min/day　My activity goal for the week: _____

My spiritual goal for the week: _____

Group	Daily Calories							
	1300-1400	1500-1600	1700-1800	1900-2000	2100-2200	2300-2400	2500-2600	2700-2800
Fruits	1.5-2 c.	1.5-2 c.	1.5-2 c.	2-2.5 c.	2-2.5 c.	2.5-3.5 c.	3.5-4.5 c.	3.5-4.5 c.
Vegetables	1.5-2 c.	2-2.5 c.	2.5-3 c.	2.5-3 c.	3-3.5 c.	3.5-4.5 c.	4.5-5 c.	4.5-5 c.
Grains	5 oz-eq.	5-6 oz-eq.	6-7 oz-eq.	6-7 oz-eq.	7-8 oz-eq.	8-9 oz-eq.	9-10 oz-eq.	10-11 oz-eq.
Meat & Beans	4 oz-eq.	5 oz-eq.	5-5.5 oz-eq.	5.5-6.5 oz-eq.	6.5-7 oz-eq.	7-7.5 oz-eq.	7-7.5 oz-eq.	7.5-8 oz-eq.
Milk	2-3 c.	3 c.	3 c.	3 c.	3 c.	3 c.	3 c.	3 c.
Healthy Oils	4 tsp.	5 tsp.	5 tsp.	6 tsp.	6 tsp.	7 tsp.	8 tsp.	8 tsp.

Day/Date:

Breakfast: _____

Lunch: _____

Dinner: _____

Snacks: _____

GROUP	FRUITS	VEGETABLES	GRAINS	MEAT & BEANS	MILK	OILS
Goal Amount						
Estimate Your Total						
Total Calories						

Physical Activity: _____　Spiritual Activity: _____

Steps/Miles/Minutes: _____　My Emotions Today: ❑ Happy　❑ Sad　❑ Stressed

Day/Date:

Breakfast: _____

Lunch: _____

Dinner: _____

Snacks: _____

GROUP	FRUITS	VEGETABLES	GRAINS	MEAT & BEANS	MILK	OILS
Goal Amount						
Estimate Your Total						
Total Calories						

Physical Activity: _____　Spiritual Activity: _____

Steps/Miles/Minutes: _____　My Emotions Today: ❑ Happy　❑ Sad　❑ Stressed

Day/Date:

Breakfast: _____

Lunch: _____

Dinner: _____

Snacks: _____

GROUP	FRUITS	VEGETABLES	GRAINS	MEAT & BEANS	MILK	OILS
Goal Amount						
Estimate Your Total						
Total Calories						

Physical Activity: _____　Spiritual Activity: _____

Steps/Miles/Minutes: _____　My Emotions Today: ❑ Happy　❑ Sad　❑ Stressed

Day/Date:

Breakfast: _____
Lunch: _____
Dinner: _____
Snacks: _____

GROUP	FRUITS	VEGETABLES	GRAINS	MEAT & BEANS	MILK	OILS
Goal Amount						
Estimate Your Total						
Total Calories						

Physical Activity: _____ Spiritual Activity: _____
Steps/Miles/Minutes: _____ My Emotions Today: ❏ Happy ❏ Sad ❏ Stressed

---

Day/Date:

Breakfast: _____
Lunch: _____
Dinner: _____
Snacks: _____

GROUP	FRUITS	VEGETABLES	GRAINS	MEAT & BEANS	MILK	OILS
Goal Amount						
Estimate Your Total						
Total Calories						

Physical Activity: _____ Spiritual Activity: _____
Steps/Miles/Minutes: _____ My Emotions Today: ❏ Happy ❏ Sad ❏ Stressed

---

Day/Date:

Breakfast: _____
Lunch: _____
Dinner: _____
Snacks: _____

GROUP	FRUITS	VEGETABLES	GRAINS	MEAT & BEANS	MILK	OILS
Goal Amount						
Estimate Your Total						
Total Calories						

Physical Activity: _____ Spiritual Activity: _____
Steps/Miles/Minutes: _____ My Emotions Today: ❏ Happy ❏ Sad ❏ Stressed

---

Day/Date:

Breakfast: _____
Lunch: _____
Dinner: _____
Snacks: _____

GROUP	FRUITS	VEGETABLES	GRAINS	MEAT & BEANS	MILK	OILS
Goal Amount						
Estimate Your Total						
Total Calories						

Physical Activity: _____ Spiritual Activity: _____
Steps/Miles/Minutes: _____ My Emotions Today: ❏ Happy ❏ Sad ❏ Stressed

Live It Tracker

Name: _____ Date: _____ Week #: _____

Loss/gain _____ lbs.   Calorie Range: _____   My food goal for the week: _____

_____

Activity Level: None, < 30 min/day, 30-60 min/day, 60+ min/day My activity goal for the week: _____

My spiritual goal for the week: _____

Group	Daily Calories							
	1300-1400	1500-1600	1700-1800	1900-2000	2100-2200	2300-2400	2500-2600	2700-2800
Fruits	1.5-2 c.	1.5-2 c.	1.5-2 c.	2-2.5 c.	2-2.5 c.	2.5-3.5 c.	3.5-4.5 c.	3.5-4.5 c.
Vegetables	1.5-2 c.	2-2.5 c.	2.5-3 c.	2.5-3 c.	3-3.5 c.	3.5-4.5 c.	4.5-5 c.	4.5-5 c.
Grains	5 oz-eq.	5-6 oz-eq.	6-7 oz-eq.	6-7 oz-eq.	7-8 oz-eq.	8-9 oz-eq.	9-10 oz-eq.	10-11 oz-eq.
Meat & Beans	4 oz-eq.	5 oz-eq.	5-5.5 oz-eq.	5.5-6.5 oz-eq.	6.5-7 oz-eq.	7-7.5 oz-eq.	7-7.5 oz-eq.	7.5-8 oz-eq.
Milk	2-3 c.	3 c.	3 c.	3 c.	3 c.	3 c.	3 c.	3 c.
Healthy Oils	4 tsp.	5 tsp.	5 tsp.	6 tsp.	6 tsp.	7 tsp.	8 tsp.	8 tsp.

Day/Date:

Breakfast: _____
Lunch: _____
Dinner: _____
Snacks: _____

GROUP	FRUITS	VEGETABLES	GRAINS	MEAT & BEANS	MILK	OILS
Goal Amount						
Estimate Your Total						
Total Calories						

Physical Activity: _____ Spiritual Activity: _____
Steps/Miles/Minutes: _____ My Emotions Today: ❑ Happy ❑ Sad ❑ Stressed

Day/Date:

Breakfast: _____
Lunch: _____
Dinner: _____
Snacks: _____

GROUP	FRUITS	VEGETABLES	GRAINS	MEAT & BEANS	MILK	OILS
Goal Amount						
Estimate Your Total						
Total Calories						

Physical Activity: _____ Spiritual Activity: _____
Steps/Miles/Minutes: _____ My Emotions Today: ❑ Happy ❑ Sad ❑ Stressed

Day/Date:

Breakfast: _____
Lunch: _____
Dinner: _____
Snacks: _____

GROUP	FRUITS	VEGETABLES	GRAINS	MEAT & BEANS	MILK	OILS
Goal Amount						
Estimate Your Total						
Total Calories						

Physical Activity: _____ Spiritual Activity: _____
Steps/Miles/Minutes: _____ My Emotions Today: ❑ Happy ❑ Sad ❑ Stressed

Breakfast: _____

Lunch: _____

Dinner: _____

Snacks: _____

GROUP	FRUITS	VEGETABLES	GRAINS	MEAT & BEANS	MILK	OILS
Goal Amount						
Estimate Your Total						
Total Calories						

Physical Activity: _____ Spiritual Activity: _____

Steps/Miles/Minutes: _____ My Emotions Today: ❑ Happy ❑ Sad ❑ Stressed

(Day/Date:)

Breakfast: _____

Lunch: _____

Dinner: _____

Snacks: _____

GROUP	FRUITS	VEGETABLES	GRAINS	MEAT & BEANS	MILK	OILS
Goal Amount						
Estimate Your Total						
Total Calories						

Physical Activity: _____ Spiritual Activity: _____

Steps/Miles/Minutes: _____ My Emotions Today: ❑ Happy ❑ Sad ❑ Stressed

(Day/Date:)

Breakfast: _____

Lunch: _____

Dinner: _____

Snacks: _____

GROUP	FRUITS	VEGETABLES	GRAINS	MEAT & BEANS	MILK	OILS
Goal Amount						
Estimate Your Total						
Total Calories						

Physical Activity: _____ Spiritual Activity: _____

Steps/Miles/Minutes: _____ My Emotions Today: ❑ Happy ❑ Sad ❑ Stressed

(Day/Date:)

Breakfast: _____

Lunch: _____

Dinner: _____

Snacks: _____

GROUP	FRUITS	VEGETABLES	GRAINS	MEAT & BEANS	MILK	OILS
Goal Amount						
Estimate Your Total						
Total Calories						

Physical Activity: _____ Spiritual Activity: _____

Steps/Miles/Minutes: _____ My Emotions Today: ❑ Happy ❑ Sad ❑ Stressed

(Day/Date:)

Live It Tracker

Name: _____ Date: _____ Week #: _____

Loss/gain _____ lbs.   Calorie Range: _____   My food goal for the week: _____

_____

Activity Level: None, < 30 min/day, 30-60 min/day, 60+ min/day My activity goal for the week: _____

My spiritual goal for the week: _____

Group	Daily Calories							
	1300-1400	1500-1600	1700-1800	1900-2000	2100-2200	2300-2400	2500-2600	2700-2800
Fruits	1.5-2 c.	1.5-2 c.	1.5-2 c.	2-2.5 c.	2-2.5 c.	2.5-3.5 c.	3.5-4.5 c.	3.5-4.5 c.
Vegetables	1.5-2 c.	2-2.5 c.	2.5-3 c.	2.5-3 c.	3-3.5 c.	3.5-4.5 c.	4.5-5 c.	4.5-5 c.
Grains	5 oz-eq.	5-6 oz-eq.	6-7 oz-eq.	6-7 oz-eq.	7-8 oz-eq.	8-9 oz-eq.	9-10 oz-eq.	10-11 oz-eq.
Meat & Beans	4 oz-eq.	5 oz-eq.	5-5.5 oz-eq.	5.5-6.5 oz-eq.	6.5-7 oz-eq.	7-7.5 oz-eq.	7-7.5 oz-eq.	7.5-8 oz-eq.
Milk	2-3 c.	3 c.	3 c.	3 c.	3 c.	3 c.	3 c.	3 c.
Healthy Oils	4 tsp.	5 tsp.	5 tsp.	6 tsp.	6 tsp.	7 tsp.	8 tsp.	8 tsp.

Day/Date:

Breakfast: _____
Lunch: _____
Dinner: _____
Snacks: _____

GROUP	FRUITS	VEGETABLES	GRAINS	MEAT & BEANS	MILK	OILS
Goal Amount						
Estimate Your Total						
Total Calories						

Physical Activity: _____ Spiritual Activity: _____
Steps/Miles/Minutes: _____ My Emotions Today: ❏ Happy ❏ Sad ❏ Stressed

Day/Date:

Breakfast: _____
Lunch: _____
Dinner: _____
Snacks: _____

GROUP	FRUITS	VEGETABLES	GRAINS	MEAT & BEANS	MILK	OILS
Goal Amount						
Estimate Your Total						
Total Calories						

Physical Activity: _____ Spiritual Activity: _____
Steps/Miles/Minutes: _____ My Emotions Today: ❏ Happy ❏ Sad ❏ Stressed

Day/Date:

Breakfast: _____
Lunch: _____
Dinner: _____
Snacks: _____

GROUP	FRUITS	VEGETABLES	GRAINS	MEAT & BEANS	MILK	OILS
Goal Amount						
Estimate Your Total						
Total Calories						

Physical Activity: _____ Spiritual Activity: _____
Steps/Miles/Minutes: _____ My Emotions Today: ❏ Happy ❏ Sad ❏ Stressed

Day/Date:

Breakfast: _____

Lunch: _____

Dinner: _____

Snacks: _____

GROUP	FRUITS	VEGETABLES	GRAINS	MEAT & BEANS	MILK	OILS
Goal Amount						
Estimate Your Total						
Total Calories						

Physical Activity: _____ Spiritual Activity: _____

Steps/Miles/Minutes: _____ My Emotions Today: ❑ Happy ❑ Sad ❑ Stressed

---

Day/Date:

Breakfast: _____

Lunch: _____

Dinner: _____

Snacks: _____

GROUP	FRUITS	VEGETABLES	GRAINS	MEAT & BEANS	MILK	OILS
Goal Amount						
Estimate Your Total						
Total Calories						

Physical Activity: _____ Spiritual Activity: _____

Steps/Miles/Minutes: _____ My Emotions Today: ❑ Happy ❑ Sad ❑ Stressed

---

Day/Date:

Breakfast: _____

Lunch: _____

Dinner: _____

Snacks: _____

GROUP	FRUITS	VEGETABLES	GRAINS	MEAT & BEANS	MILK	OILS
Goal Amount						
Estimate Your Total						
Total Calories						

Physical Activity: _____ Spiritual Activity: _____

Steps/Miles/Minutes: _____ My Emotions Today: ❑ Happy ❑ Sad ❑ Stressed

---

Day/Date:

Breakfast: _____

Lunch: _____

Dinner: _____

Snacks: _____

GROUP	FRUITS	VEGETABLES	GRAINS	MEAT & BEANS	MILK	OILS
Goal Amount						
Estimate Your Total						
Total Calories						

Physical Activity: _____ Spiritual Activity: _____

Steps/Miles/Minutes: _____ My Emotions Today: ❑ Happy ❑ Sad ❑ Stressed

Live It Tracker

Name: _____ Date: _____ Week #: _____

Loss/gain _____ lbs.   Calorie Range: _____   My food goal for the week: _____

_____

Activity Level: None, < 30 min/day, 30-60 min/day, 60+ min/day My activity goal for the week: _____

My spiritual goal for the week: _____

Group	Daily Calories							
	1300-1400	1500-1600	1700-1800	1900-2000	2100-2200	2300-2400	2500-2600	2700-2800
Fruits	1.5-2 c.	1.5-2 c.	1.5-2 c.	2-2.5 c.	2-2.5 c.	2.5-3.5 c.	3.5-4.5 c.	3.5-4.5 c.
Vegetables	1.5-2 c.	2-2.5 c.	2.5-3 c.	2.5-3 c.	3-3.5 c.	3.5-4.5 c.	4.5-5 c.	4.5-5 c.
Grains	5 oz-eq.	5-6 oz-eq.	6-7 oz-eq.	6-7 oz-eq.	7-8 oz-eq.	8-9 oz-eq.	9-10 oz-eq.	10-11 oz-eq.
Meat & Beans	4 oz-eq.	5 oz-eq.	5-5.5 oz-eq.	5.5-6.5 oz-eq.	6.5-7 oz-eq.	7-7.5 oz-eq.	7-7.5 oz-eq.	7.5-8 oz-eq.
Milk	2-3 c.	3 c.	3 c.	3 c.	3 c.	3 c.	3 c.	3 c.
Healthy Oils	4 tsp.	5 tsp.	5 tsp.	6 tsp.	6 tsp.	7 tsp.	8 tsp.	8 tsp.

Day/Date:

Breakfast: _____

Lunch: _____

Dinner: _____

Snacks: _____

GROUP	FRUITS	VEGETABLES	GRAINS	MEAT & BEANS	MILK	OILS
Goal Amount						
Estimate Your Total						
Total Calories						

Physical Activity: _____   Spiritual Activity: _____

Steps/Miles/Minutes: _____   My Emotions Today: ❏ Happy   ❏ Sad   ❏ Stressed

Day/Date:

Breakfast: _____

Lunch: _____

Dinner: _____

Snacks: _____

GROUP	FRUITS	VEGETABLES	GRAINS	MEAT & BEANS	MILK	OILS
Goal Amount						
Estimate Your Total						
Total Calories						

Physical Activity: _____   Spiritual Activity: _____

Steps/Miles/Minutes: _____   My Emotions Today: ❏ Happy   ❏ Sad   ❏ Stressed

Day/Date:

Breakfast: _____

Lunch: _____

Dinner: _____

Snacks: _____

GROUP	FRUITS	VEGETABLES	GRAINS	MEAT & BEANS	MILK	OILS
Goal Amount						
Estimate Your Total						
Total Calories						

Physical Activity: _____   Spiritual Activity: _____

Steps/Miles/Minutes: _____   My Emotions Today: ❏ Happy   ❏ Sad   ❏ Stressed

Day/Date: _____

Breakfast: _____
Lunch: _____
Dinner: _____
Snacks: _____

GROUP	FRUITS	VEGETABLES	GRAINS	MEAT & BEANS	MILK	OILS
Goal Amount						
Estimate Your Total						
Total Calories						

Physical Activity: _____ Spiritual Activity: _____
Steps/Miles/Minutes: _____ My Emotions Today: ❑ Happy ❑ Sad ❑ Stressed

---

Day/Date: _____

Breakfast: _____
Lunch: _____
Dinner: _____
Snacks: _____

GROUP	FRUITS	VEGETABLES	GRAINS	MEAT & BEANS	MILK	OILS
Goal Amount						
Estimate Your Total						
Total Calories						

Physical Activity: _____ Spiritual Activity: _____
Steps/Miles/Minutes: _____ My Emotions Today: ❑ Happy ❑ Sad ❑ Stressed

---

Day/Date: _____

Breakfast: _____
Lunch: _____
Dinner: _____
Snacks: _____

GROUP	FRUITS	VEGETABLES	GRAINS	MEAT & BEANS	MILK	OILS
Goal Amount						
Estimate Your Total						
Total Calories						

Physical Activity: _____ Spiritual Activity: _____
Steps/Miles/Minutes: _____ My Emotions Today: ❑ Happy ❑ Sad ❑ Stressed

---

Day/Date: _____

Breakfast: _____
Lunch: _____
Dinner: _____
Snacks: _____

GROUP	FRUITS	VEGETABLES	GRAINS	MEAT & BEANS	MILK	OILS
Goal Amount						
Estimate Your Total						
Total Calories						

Physical Activity: _____ Spiritual Activity: _____
Steps/Miles/Minutes: _____ My Emotions Today: ❑ Happy ❑ Sad ❑ Stressed

Live It Tracker

Name: _____ Date: _____ Week #: _____

Loss/gain _____ lbs.   Calorie Range: _____   My food goal for the week: _____

_____

Activity Level: None, < 30 min/day, 30-60 min/day, 60+ min/day My activity goal for the week: _____

My spiritual goal for the week: _____

Group	Daily Calories							
	1300-1400	1500-1600	1700-1800	1900-2000	2100-2200	2300-2400	2500-2600	2700-2800
Fruits	1.5-2 c.	1.5-2 c.	1.5-2 c.	2-2.5 c.	2-2.5 c.	2.5-3.5 c.	3.5-4.5 c.	3.5-4.5 c.
Vegetables	1.5-2 c.	2-2.5 c.	2.5-3 c.	2.5-3 c.	3-3.5 c.	3.5-4.5 c.	4.5-5 c.	4.5-5 c.
Grains	5 oz-eq.	5-6 oz-eq.	6-7 oz-eq.	6-7 oz-eq.	7-8 oz-eq.	8-9 oz-eq.	9-10 oz-eq.	10-11 oz-eq.
Meat & Beans	4 oz-eq.	5 oz-eq.	5-5.5 oz-eq.	5.5-6.5 oz-eq.	6.5-7 oz-eq.	7-7.5 oz-eq.	7-7.5 oz-eq.	7.5-8 oz-eq.
Milk	2-3 c.	3 c.	3 c.	3 c.	3 c.	3 c.	3 c.	3 c.
Healthy Oils	4 tsp.	5 tsp.	5 tsp.	6 tsp.	6 tsp.	7 tsp.	8 tsp.	8 tsp.

Day/Date:

Breakfast: _____
Lunch: _____
Dinner: _____
Snacks: _____

GROUP	FRUITS	VEGETABLES	GRAINS	MEAT & BEANS	MILK	OILS
Goal Amount						
Estimate Your Total						
Total Calories						

Physical Activity: _____ Spiritual Activity: _____
Steps/Miles/Minutes: _____ My Emotions Today: ❏ Happy   ❏ Sad   ❏ Stressed

Day/Date:

Breakfast: _____
Lunch: _____
Dinner: _____
Snacks: _____

GROUP	FRUITS	VEGETABLES	GRAINS	MEAT & BEANS	MILK	OILS
Goal Amount						
Estimate Your Total						
Total Calories						

Physical Activity: _____ Spiritual Activity: _____
Steps/Miles/Minutes: _____ My Emotions Today: ❏ Happy   ❏ Sad   ❏ Stressed

Day/Date:

Breakfast: _____
Lunch: _____
Dinner: _____
Snacks: _____

GROUP	FRUITS	VEGETABLES	GRAINS	MEAT & BEANS	MILK	OILS
Goal Amount						
Estimate Your Total						
Total Calories						

Physical Activity: _____ Spiritual Activity: _____
Steps/Miles/Minutes: _____ My Emotions Today: ❏ Happy   ❏ Sad   ❏ Stressed

Day/Date:

Breakfast: _____

Lunch: _____

Dinner: _____

Snacks: _____

GROUP	FRUITS	VEGETABLES	GRAINS	MEAT & BEANS	MILK	OILS
Goal Amount						
Estimate Your Total						
Total Calories						

Physical Activity: _____ Spiritual Activity: _____

Steps/Miles/Minutes: _____ My Emotions Today: ❑ Happy ❑ Sad ❑ Stressed

---

Day/Date:

Breakfast: _____

Lunch: _____

Dinner: _____

Snacks: _____

GROUP	FRUITS	VEGETABLES	GRAINS	MEAT & BEANS	MILK	OILS
Goal Amount						
Estimate Your Total						
Total Calories						

Physical Activity: _____ Spiritual Activity: _____

Steps/Miles/Minutes: _____ My Emotions Today: ❑ Happy ❑ Sad ❑ Stressed

---

Day/Date:

Breakfast: _____

Lunch: _____

Dinner: _____

Snacks: _____

GROUP	FRUITS	VEGETABLES	GRAINS	MEAT & BEANS	MILK	OILS
Goal Amount						
Estimate Your Total						
Total Calories						

Physical Activity: _____ Spiritual Activity: _____

Steps/Miles/Minutes: _____ My Emotions Today: ❑ Happy ❑ Sad ❑ Stressed

---

Day/Date:

Breakfast: _____

Lunch: _____

Dinner: _____

Snacks: _____

GROUP	FRUITS	VEGETABLES	GRAINS	MEAT & BEANS	MILK	OILS
Goal Amount						
Estimate Your Total						
Total Calories						

Physical Activity: _____ Spiritual Activity: _____

Steps/Miles/Minutes: _____ My Emotions Today: ❑ Happy ❑ Sad ❑ Stressed

Live It Tracker

Name: _____ Date: _____ Week #: _____

Loss/gain _____ lbs. Calorie Range: _____ My food goal for the week: _____

_____

Activity Level: None, < 30 min/day, 30-60 min/day, 60+ min/day My activity goal for the week: _____

My spiritual goal for the week: _____

Group	Daily Calories							
	1300-1400	1500-1600	1700-1800	1900-2000	2100-2200	2300-2400	2500-2600	2700-2800
Fruits	1.5-2 c.	1.5-2 c.	1.5-2 c.	2-2.5 c.	2-2.5 c.	2.5-3.5 c.	3.5-4.5 c.	3.5-4.5 c.
Vegetables	1.5-2 c.	2-2.5 c.	2.5-3 c.	2.5-3 c.	3-3.5 c.	3.5-4.5 c.	4.5-5 c.	4.5-5 c.
Grains	5 oz-eq.	5-6 oz-eq.	6-7 oz-eq.	6-7 oz-eq.	7-8 oz-eq.	8-9 oz-eq.	9-10 oz-eq.	10-11 oz-eq.
Meat & Beans	4 oz-eq.	5 oz-eq.	5-5.5 oz-eq.	5.5-6.5 oz-eq.	6.5-7 oz-eq.	7-7.5 oz-eq.	7-7.5 oz-eq.	7.5-8 oz-eq.
Milk	2-3 c.	3 c.	3 c.	3 c.	3 c.	3 c.	3 c.	3 c.
Healthy Oils	4 tsp.	5 tsp.	5 tsp.	6 tsp.	6 tsp.	7 tsp.	8 tsp.	8 tsp.

Day/Date:

Breakfast: _____
Lunch: _____
Dinner: _____
Snacks: _____

GROUP	FRUITS	VEGETABLES	GRAINS	MEAT & BEANS	MILK	OILS
Goal Amount						
Estimate Your Total						
Total Calories						

Physical Activity: _____ Spiritual Activity: _____
Steps/Miles/Minutes: _____ My Emotions Today: ❑ Happy ❑ Sad ❑ Stressed

Day/Date:

Breakfast: _____
Lunch: _____
Dinner: _____
Snacks: _____

GROUP	FRUITS	VEGETABLES	GRAINS	MEAT & BEANS	MILK	OILS
Goal Amount						
Estimate Your Total						
Total Calories						

Physical Activity: _____ Spiritual Activity: _____
Steps/Miles/Minutes: _____ My Emotions Today: ❑ Happy ❑ Sad ❑ Stressed

Day/Date:

Breakfast: _____
Lunch: _____
Dinner: _____
Snacks: _____

GROUP	FRUITS	VEGETABLES	GRAINS	MEAT & BEANS	MILK	OILS
Goal Amount						
Estimate Your Total						
Total Calories						

Physical Activity: _____ Spiritual Activity: _____
Steps/Miles/Minutes: _____ My Emotions Today: ❑ Happy ❑ Sad ❑ Stressed

Day/Date:

Breakfast: _____
Lunch: _____
Dinner: _____
Snacks: _____

GROUP	FRUITS	VEGETABLES	GRAINS	MEAT & BEANS	MILK	OILS
Goal Amount						
Estimate Your Total						
Total Calories						

Physical Activity: _____   Spiritual Activity: _____

Steps/Miles/Minutes: _____   My Emotions Today: ❑ Happy   ❑ Sad   ❑ Stressed

---

Day/Date:

Breakfast: _____
Lunch: _____
Dinner: _____
Snacks: _____

GROUP	FRUITS	VEGETABLES	GRAINS	MEAT & BEANS	MILK	OILS
Goal Amount						
Estimate Your Total						
Total Calories						

Physical Activity: _____   Spiritual Activity: _____

Steps/Miles/Minutes: _____   My Emotions Today: ❑ Happy   ❑ Sad   ❑ Stressed

---

Day/Date:

Breakfast: _____
Lunch: _____
Dinner: _____
Snacks: _____

GROUP	FRUITS	VEGETABLES	GRAINS	MEAT & BEANS	MILK	OILS
Goal Amount						
Estimate Your Total						
Total Calories						

Physical Activity: _____   Spiritual Activity: _____

Steps/Miles/Minutes: _____   My Emotions Today: ❑ Happy   ❑ Sad   ❑ Stressed

---

Day/Date:

Breakfast: _____
Lunch: _____
Dinner: _____
Snacks: _____

GROUP	FRUITS	VEGETABLES	GRAINS	MEAT & BEANS	MILK	OILS
Goal Amount						
Estimate Your Total						
Total Calories						

Physical Activity: _____   Spiritual Activity: _____

Steps/Miles/Minutes: _____   My Emotions Today: ❑ Happy   ❑ Sad   ❑ Stressed

Live It Tracker

Name: _____ Date: _____ Week #: _____

Loss/gain _____ lbs. Calorie Range: _____ My food goal for the week: _____
_____

Activity Level: None, < 30 min/day, 30-60 min/day, 60+ min/day My activity goal for the week: _____

My spiritual goal for the week: _____

Group	Daily Calories							
	1300-1400	1500-1600	1700-1800	1900-2000	2100-2200	2300-2400	2500-2600	2700-2800
Fruits	1.5-2 c.	1.5-2 c.	1.5-2 c.	2-2.5 c.	2-2.5 c.	2.5-3.5 c.	3.5-4.5 c.	3.5-4.5 c.
Vegetables	1.5-2 c.	2-2.5 c.	2.5-3 c.	2.5-3 c.	3-3.5 c.	3.5-4.5 c.	4.5-5 c.	4.5-5 c.
Grains	5 oz-eq.	5-6 oz-eq.	6-7 oz-eq.	6-7 oz-eq.	7-8 oz-eq.	8-9 oz-eq.	9-10 oz-eq.	10-11 oz-eq.
Meat & Beans	4 oz-eq.	5 oz-eq.	5-5.5 oz-eq.	5.5-6.5 oz-eq.	6.5-7 oz-eq.	7-7.5 oz-eq.	7-7.5 oz-eq.	7.5-8 oz-eq.
Milk	2-3 c.	3 c.	3 c.	3 c.	3 c.	3 c.	3 c.	3 c.
Healthy Oils	4 tsp.	5 tsp.	5 tsp.	6 tsp.	6 tsp.	7 tsp.	8 tsp.	8 tsp.

Day/Date:

Breakfast: _____
Lunch: _____
Dinner: _____
Snacks: _____

GROUP	FRUITS	VEGETABLES	GRAINS	MEAT & BEANS	MILK	OILS
Goal Amount						
Estimate Your Total						
Total Calories						

Physical Activity: _____ Spiritual Activity: _____
Steps/Miles/Minutes: _____ My Emotions Today: ❏ Happy ❏ Sad ❏ Stressed

Day/Date:

Breakfast: _____
Lunch: _____
Dinner: _____
Snacks: _____

GROUP	FRUITS	VEGETABLES	GRAINS	MEAT & BEANS	MILK	OILS
Goal Amount						
Estimate Your Total						
Total Calories						

Physical Activity: _____ Spiritual Activity: _____
Steps/Miles/Minutes: _____ My Emotions Today: ❏ Happy ❏ Sad ❏ Stressed

Day/Date:

Breakfast: _____
Lunch: _____
Dinner: _____
Snacks: _____

GROUP	FRUITS	VEGETABLES	GRAINS	MEAT & BEANS	MILK	OILS
Goal Amount						
Estimate Your Total						
Total Calories						

Physical Activity: _____ Spiritual Activity: _____
Steps/Miles/Minutes: _____ My Emotions Today: ❏ Happy ❏ Sad ❏ Stressed

Day/Date:

Breakfast: _____

Lunch: _____

Dinner: _____

Snacks: _____

GROUP	FRUITS	VEGETABLES	GRAINS	MEAT & BEANS	MILK	OILS
Goal Amount						
Estimate Your Total						
Total Calories						

Physical Activity: _____

Steps/Miles/Minutes: _____

Spiritual Activity: _____

My Emotions Today: ❑ Happy ❑ Sad ❑ Stressed

Day/Date:

Breakfast: _____

Lunch: _____

Dinner: _____

Snacks: _____

GROUP	FRUITS	VEGETABLES	GRAINS	MEAT & BEANS	MILK	OILS
Goal Amount						
Estimate Your Total						
Total Calories						

Physical Activity: _____

Steps/Miles/Minutes: _____

Spiritual Activity: _____

My Emotions Today: ❑ Happy ❑ Sad ❑ Stressed

Day/Date:

Breakfast: _____

Lunch: _____

Dinner: _____

Snacks: _____

GROUP	FRUITS	VEGETABLES	GRAINS	MEAT & BEANS	MILK	OILS
Goal Amount						
Estimate Your Total						
Total Calories						

Physical Activity: _____

Steps/Miles/Minutes: _____

Spiritual Activity: _____

My Emotions Today: ❑ Happy ❑ Sad ❑ Stressed

Day/Date:

Breakfast: _____

Lunch: _____

Dinner: _____

Snacks: _____

GROUP	FRUITS	VEGETABLES	GRAINS	MEAT & BEANS	MILK	OILS
Goal Amount						
Estimate Your Total						
Total Calories						

Physical Activity: _____

Steps/Miles/Minutes: _____

Spiritual Activity: _____

My Emotions Today: ❑ Happy ❑ Sad ❑ Stressed

Live It Tracker

Name: _____ Date: _____ Week #: _____

Loss/gain _____ lbs.   Calorie Range: _____   My food goal for the week: _____
_____

Activity Level: None, < 30 min/day, 30-60 min/day, 60+ min/day My activity goal for the week: _____
My spiritual goal for the week: _____

Group	Daily Calories							
	1300-1400	1500-1600	1700-1800	1900-2000	2100-2200	2300-2400	2500-2600	2700-2800
Fruits	1.5-2 c.	1.5-2 c.	1.5-2 c.	2-2.5 c.	2-2.5 c.	2.5-3.5 c.	3.5-4.5 c.	3.5-4.5 c.
Vegetables	1.5-2 c.	2-2.5 c.	2.5-3 c.	2.5-3 c.	3-3.5 c.	3.5-4.5 c.	4.5-5 c.	4.5-5 c.
Grains	5 oz-eq.	5-6 oz-eq.	6-7 oz-eq.	6-7 oz-eq.	7-8 oz-eq.	8-9 oz-eq.	9-10 oz-eq.	10-11 oz-eq.
Meat & Beans	4 oz-eq.	5 oz-eq.	5-5.5 oz-eq.	5.5-6.5 oz-eq.	6.5-7 oz-eq.	7-7.5 oz-eq.	7-7.5 oz-eq.	7.5-8 oz-eq.
Milk	2-3 c.	3 c.	3 c.	3 c.	3 c.	3 c.	3 c.	3 c.
Healthy Oils	4 tsp.	5 tsp.	5 tsp.	6 tsp.	6 tsp.	7 tsp.	8 tsp.	8 tsp.

Day/Date:

Breakfast: _____
Lunch: _____
Dinner: _____
Snacks: _____

GROUP	FRUITS	VEGETABLES	GRAINS	MEAT & BEANS	MILK	OILS
Goal Amount						
Estimate Your Total						
Total Calories						

Physical Activity: _____   Spiritual Activity: _____
Steps/Miles/Minutes: _____   My Emotions Today: ❑ Happy ❑ Sad ❑ Stressed

Day/Date:

Breakfast: _____
Lunch: _____
Dinner: _____
Snacks: _____

GROUP	FRUITS	VEGETABLES	GRAINS	MEAT & BEANS	MILK	OILS
Goal Amount						
Estimate Your Total						
Total Calories						

Physical Activity: _____   Spiritual Activity: _____
Steps/Miles/Minutes: _____   My Emotions Today: ❑ Happy ❑ Sad ❑ Stressed

Day/Date:

Breakfast: _____
Lunch: _____
Dinner: _____
Snacks: _____

GROUP	FRUITS	VEGETABLES	GRAINS	MEAT & BEANS	MILK	OILS
Goal Amount						
Estimate Your Total						
Total Calories						

Physical Activity: _____   Spiritual Activity: _____
Steps/Miles/Minutes: _____   My Emotions Today: ❑ Happy ❑ Sad ❑ Stressed

Day/Date: ______

Breakfast:

Lunch:

Dinner:

Snacks:

GROUP	FRUITS	VEGETABLES	GRAINS	MEAT & BEANS	MILK	OILS
Goal Amount						
Estimate Your Total						
Total Calories						

Physical Activity:

Spiritual Activity:

Steps/Miles/Minutes:

My Emotions Today: ❑ Happy ❑ Sad ❑ Stressed

Day/Date: ______

Breakfast:

Lunch:

Dinner:

Snacks:

GROUP	FRUITS	VEGETABLES	GRAINS	MEAT & BEANS	MILK	OILS
Goal Amount						
Estimate Your Total						
Total Calories						

Physical Activity:

Spiritual Activity:

Steps/Miles/Minutes:

My Emotions Today: ❑ Happy ❑ Sad ❑ Stressed

Day/Date: ______

Breakfast:

Lunch:

Dinner:

Snacks:

GROUP	FRUITS	VEGETABLES	GRAINS	MEAT & BEANS	MILK	OILS
Goal Amount						
Estimate Your Total						
Total Calories						

Physical Activity:

Spiritual Activity:

Steps/Miles/Minutes:

My Emotions Today: ❑ Happy ❑ Sad ❑ Stressed

Day/Date: ______

Breakfast:

Lunch:

Dinner:

Snacks:

GROUP	FRUITS	VEGETABLES	GRAINS	MEAT & BEANS	MILK	OILS
Goal Amount						
Estimate Your Total						
Total Calories						

Physical Activity:

Spiritual Activity:

Steps/Miles/Minutes:

My Emotions Today: ❑ Happy ❑ Sad ❑ Stressed

Live It Tracker

Name: _____ Date: _____ Week #: _____

Loss/gain _____ lbs.   Calorie Range: _____   My food goal for the week: _____

Activity Level: None, < 30 min/day, 30-60 min/day, 60+ min/day My activity goal for the week: _____

My spiritual goal for the week: _____

Group	Daily Calories							
	1300-1400	1500-1600	1700-1800	1900-2000	2100-2200	2300-2400	2500-2600	2700-2800
Fruits	1.5-2 c.	1.5-2 c.	1.5-2 c.	2-2.5 c.	2-2.5 c.	2.5-3.5 c.	3.5-4.5 c.	3.5-4.5 c.
Vegetables	1.5-2 c.	2-2.5 c.	2.5-3 c.	2.5-3 c.	3-3.5 c.	3.5-4.5 c.	4.5-5 c.	4.5-5 c.
Grains	5 oz-eq.	5-6 oz-eq.	6-7 oz-eq.	6-7 oz-eq.	7-8 oz-eq.	8-9 oz-eq.	9-10 oz-eq.	10-11 oz-eq.
Meat & Beans	4 oz-eq.	5 oz-eq.	5-5.5 oz-eq.	5.5-6.5 oz-eq.	6.5-7 oz-eq.	7-7.5 oz-eq.	7-7.5 oz-eq.	7.5-8 oz-eq.
Milk	2-3 c.	3 c.	3 c.	3 c.	3 c.	3 c.	3 c.	3 c.
Healthy Oils	4 tsp.	5 tsp.	5 tsp.	6 tsp.	6 tsp.	7 tsp.	8 tsp.	8 tsp.

Day/Date:

Breakfast: _____
Lunch: _____
Dinner: _____
Snacks: _____

GROUP	FRUITS	VEGETABLES	GRAINS	MEAT & BEANS	MILK	OILS
Goal Amount						
Estimate Your Total						
Total Calories						

Physical Activity: _____ Spiritual Activity: _____
Steps/Miles/Minutes: _____ My Emotions Today: ❑ Happy ❑ Sad ❑ Stressed

Day/Date:

Breakfast: _____
Lunch: _____
Dinner: _____
Snacks: _____

GROUP	FRUITS	VEGETABLES	GRAINS	MEAT & BEANS	MILK	OILS
Goal Amount						
Estimate Your Total						
Total Calories						

Physical Activity: _____ Spiritual Activity: _____
Steps/Miles/Minutes: _____ My Emotions Today: ❑ Happy ❑ Sad ❑ Stressed

Day/Date:

Breakfast: _____
Lunch: _____
Dinner: _____
Snacks: _____

GROUP	FRUITS	VEGETABLES	GRAINS	MEAT & BEANS	MILK	OILS
Goal Amount						
Estimate Your Total						
Total Calories						

Physical Activity: _____ Spiritual Activity: _____
Steps/Miles/Minutes: _____ My Emotions Today: ❑ Happy ❑ Sad ❑ Stressed

Day/Date:

Breakfast: _____
Lunch: _____
Dinner: _____
Snacks: _____

GROUP	FRUITS	VEGETABLES	GRAINS	MEAT & BEANS	MILK	OILS
Goal Amount						
Estimate Your Total						
Total Calories						

Physical Activity: _____   Spiritual Activity: _____
Steps/Miles/Minutes: _____   My Emotions Today: ❑ Happy ❑ Sad ❑ Stressed

---

Day/Date:

Breakfast: _____
Lunch: _____
Dinner: _____
Snacks: _____

GROUP	FRUITS	VEGETABLES	GRAINS	MEAT & BEANS	MILK	OILS
Goal Amount						
Estimate Your Total						
Total Calories						

Physical Activity: _____   Spiritual Activity: _____
Steps/Miles/Minutes: _____   My Emotions Today: ❑ Happy ❑ Sad ❑ Stressed

---

Day/Date:

Breakfast: _____
Lunch: _____
Dinner: _____
Snacks: _____

GROUP	FRUITS	VEGETABLES	GRAINS	MEAT & BEANS	MILK	OILS
Goal Amount						
Estimate Your Total						
Total Calories						

Physical Activity: _____   Spiritual Activity: _____
Steps/Miles/Minutes: _____   My Emotions Today: ❑ Happy ❑ Sad ❑ Stressed

---

Day/Date:

Breakfast: _____
Lunch: _____
Dinner: _____
Snacks: _____

GROUP	FRUITS	VEGETABLES	GRAINS	MEAT & BEANS	MILK	OILS
Goal Amount						
Estimate Your Total						
Total Calories						

Physical Activity: _____   Spiritual Activity: _____
Steps/Miles/Minutes: _____   My Emotions Today: ❑ Happy ❑ Sad ❑ Stressed

Live It Tracker

Name: _____ Date: _____ Week #: _____

Loss/gain _____ lbs.   Calorie Range: _____   My food goal for the week: _____

_____

Activity Level: None, < 30 min/day, 30-60 min/day, 60+ min/day My activity goal for the week: _____

My spiritual goal for the week: _____

Group	Daily Calories							
	1300-1400	1500-1600	1700-1800	1900-2000	2100-2200	2300-2400	2500-2600	2700-2800
Fruits	1.5-2 c.	1.5-2 c.	1.5-2 c.	2-2.5 c.	2-2.5 c.	2.5-3.5 c.	3.5-4.5 c.	3.5-4.5 c.
Vegetables	1.5-2 c.	2-2.5 c.	2.5-3 c.	2.5-3 c.	3-3.5 c.	3.5-4.5 c.	4.5-5 c.	4.5-5 c.
Grains	5 oz-eq.	5-6 oz-eq.	6-7 oz-eq.	6-7 oz-eq.	7-8 oz-eq.	8-9 oz-eq.	9-10 oz-eq.	10-11 oz-eq.
Meat & Beans	4 oz-eq.	5 oz-eq.	5-5.5 oz-eq.	5.5-6.5 oz-eq.	6.5-7 oz-eq.	7-7.5 oz-eq.	7-7.5 oz-eq.	7.5-8 oz-eq.
Milk	2-3 c.	3 c.	3 c.	3 c.	3 c.	3 c.	3 c.	3 c.
Healthy Oils	4 tsp.	5 tsp.	5 tsp.	6 tsp.	6 tsp.	7 tsp.	8 tsp.	8 tsp.

Day/Date:

Breakfast: _____

Lunch: _____

Dinner: _____

Snacks: _____

GROUP	FRUITS	VEGETABLES	GRAINS	MEAT & BEANS	MILK	OILS
Goal Amount						
Estimate Your Total						
Total Calories						

Physical Activity: _____   Spiritual Activity: _____

Steps/Miles/Minutes: _____   My Emotions Today: ❏ Happy   ❏ Sad   ❏ Stressed

Day/Date:

Breakfast: _____

Lunch: _____

Dinner: _____

Snacks: _____

GROUP	FRUITS	VEGETABLES	GRAINS	MEAT & BEANS	MILK	OILS
Goal Amount						
Estimate Your Total						
Total Calories						

Physical Activity: _____   Spiritual Activity: _____

Steps/Miles/Minutes: _____   My Emotions Today: ❏ Happy   ❏ Sad   ❏ Stressed

Day/Date:

Breakfast: _____

Lunch: _____

Dinner: _____

Snacks: _____

GROUP	FRUITS	VEGETABLES	GRAINS	MEAT & BEANS	MILK	OILS
Goal Amount						
Estimate Your Total						
Total Calories						

Physical Activity: _____   Spiritual Activity: _____

Steps/Miles/Minutes: _____   My Emotions Today: ❏ Happy   ❏ Sad   ❏ Stressed

Day/Date:

Breakfast: _____
Lunch: _____
Dinner: _____
Snacks: _____

GROUP	FRUITS	VEGETABLES	GRAINS	MEAT & BEANS	MILK	OILS
Goal Amount						
Estimate Your Total						
Total Calories						

Physical Activity: _____ Spiritual Activity: _____
Steps/Miles/Minutes: _____ My Emotions Today: ❑ Happy ❑ Sad ❑ Stressed

---

Day/Date:

Breakfast: _____
Lunch: _____
Dinner: _____
Snacks: _____

GROUP	FRUITS	VEGETABLES	GRAINS	MEAT & BEANS	MILK	OILS
Goal Amount						
Estimate Your Total						
Total Calories						

Physical Activity: _____ Spiritual Activity: _____
Steps/Miles/Minutes: _____ My Emotions Today: ❑ Happy ❑ Sad ❑ Stressed

---

Day/Date:

Breakfast: _____
Lunch: _____
Dinner: _____
Snacks: _____

GROUP	FRUITS	VEGETABLES	GRAINS	MEAT & BEANS	MILK	OILS
Goal Amount						
Estimate Your Total						
Total Calories						

Physical Activity: _____ Spiritual Activity: _____
Steps/Miles/Minutes: _____ My Emotions Today: ❑ Happy ❑ Sad ❑ Stressed

---

Day/Date:

Breakfast: _____
Lunch: _____
Dinner: _____
Snacks: _____

GROUP	FRUITS	VEGETABLES	GRAINS	MEAT & BEANS	MILK	OILS
Goal Amount						
Estimate Your Total						
Total Calories						

Physical Activity: _____ Spiritual Activity: _____
Steps/Miles/Minutes: _____ My Emotions Today: ❑ Happy ❑ Sad ❑ Stressed

let's count our miles!

Join the 100-Mile Club this Session

Can't walk that mile yet? Don't be discouraged! There are exercises you can do to strengthen your body and burn those extra calories. Keep a record on your Live It Tracker of the number of minutes you do these common physical activities, convert those minutes to miles following the chart below, and then mark off each mile you have completed on the chart found on the back of the back cover. Report your miles to your 100-Mile Club representative when you first arrive each week. Remember, you are not competing with anyone else . . . just yourself. Your job is to strive to reach 100 miles before the last meeting in this session. You can do it—just keep on moving!

Walking

slowly, 2 mph	30 min. = 156 cal. = 1 mile
moderately, 3 mph	20 min. = 156 cal. = 1 mile
very briskly, 4 mph	15 min. = 156 cal. = 1 mile
speed walking	10 min. = 156 cal. = 1 mile
up stairs	13 min. = 159 cal. = 1 mile

Running/Jogging

10 min. = 156 cal. = 1 mile

Cycling Outdoors

slowly, <10 mph	20 min. = 156 cal. = 1 mile
light effort, 10-12 mph	12 min. = 156 cal. = 1 mile
moderate effort, 12-14 mph	10 min. = 156 cal. = 1 mile
vigorous effort, 14-16 mph	7.5 min. = 156 cal. = 1 mile
very fast, 16-19 mph	6.5 min. = 152 cal. = 1 mile

Sports Activities

Playing tennis (singles)	10 min. = 156 cal. = 1 mile
Swimming	
light to moderate effort	11 min. = 152 cal. = 1 mile
fast, vigorous effort	7.5 min. = 156 cal. = 1 mile
Softball	15 min. = 156 cal. = 1 mile
Golf	20 min. = 156 cal = 1 mile
Rollerblading	6.5 min. = 152 cal. = 1 mile
Ice skating	11 min. = 152 cal. = 1 mile

Jumping rope	7.5 min. = 156 cal. = 1 mile
Basketball	12 min. = 156 cal. = 1 mile
Soccer (casual)	15 min. = 159 cal. = 1 mile

Around the House

Mowing grass	22 min. = 156 cal. = 1 mile
Mopping, sweeping, vacuuming	19.5 min. = 155 cal. = 1 mile
Cooking	40 min. =160 cal. = 1 mile
Gardening	19 min. = 156 cal. = 1 mile
Housework (general)	35 min. = 156 cal. = 1 mile
Ironing	45 min. = 153 cal. = 1 mile
Raking leaves	25 min. = 150 cal. = 1 mile
Washing car	23 min. = 156 cal. = 1 mile
Washing dishes	45 min. = 153 cal. = 1 mile

At the Gym

Stair machine	8.5 min. = 155 cal. = 1 mile
Stationary bike	
slowly, 10 mph	30 min. = 156 cal. = 1 mile
moderately, 10-13 mph	15 min. = 156 cal. = 1 mile
vigorously, 13-16 mph	7.5 min. = 156 cal. = 1 mile
briskly, 16-19 mph	6.5 min. = 156 cal. = 1 mile
Elliptical trainer	12 min. = 156 cal. = 1 mile
Weight machines (used vigorously)	13 min. = 152 cal.=1 mile
Aerobics	
low impact	15 min. = 156 cal. = 1 mile
high impact	12 min. = 156 cal. = 1 mile
water	20 min. = 156 cal. = 1 mile
Pilates	15 min. = 156 cal. = 1 mile
Raquetball (casual)	15 min. = 159 cal. = 1 mile
Stretching exercises	25 min. = 150 cal. = 1 mile
Weight lifting (also works for weight machines used moderately or gently)	30 min. = 156 cal. = 1 mile

Family Leisure

Playing piano	37 min. = 155 cal. = 1 mile
Jumping rope	10 min. = 152 cal. = 1 mile
Skating (moderate)	20 min. = 152 cal. = 1 mile
Swimming	
moderate	17 min. = 156 cal. = 1 mile
vigorous	10 min. = 148 cal. = 1 mile
Table tennis	25 min. = 150 cal. = 1 mile
Walk/run/play with kids	25 min. = 150 cal. = 1 mile